CM01602335

Ten things I wish you knew about your child's mental health

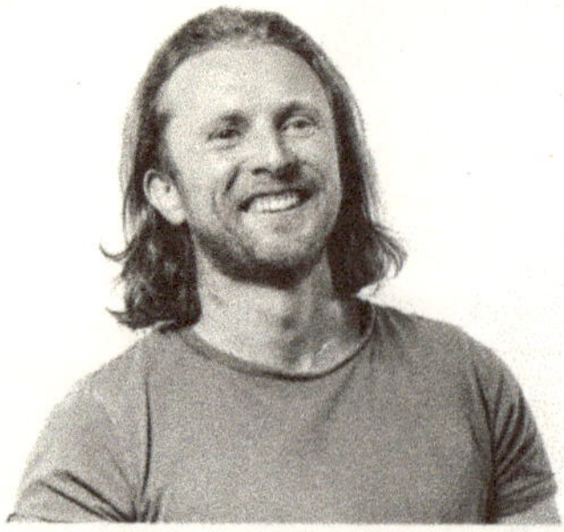

Dr Billy Garvey is a developmental paediatrician with over 20 years' experience working with children. He is a senior specialist at one of the largest tertiary paediatric hospitals in the world, where he sees families, trains clinicians and other professionals working with children and conducts research in child development and mental health. He is also the founder of Guiding Growing Minds, a social enterprise that aims to give all children the opportunity to reach their potential and live rich and meaningful lives. The Pop Culture Parenting podcast is a part of this vision.

Ten things I wish you knew about your child's mental health

Dr BILLY GARVEY

LIFE

PENGUIN LIFE

UK | USA | Canada | Ireland | Australia
India | New Zealand | South Africa | China

Penguin Life is part of the Penguin Random House group of companies whose addresses can be found at global.penguinrandomhouse.com.

Penguin Random House Australia

First published by Penguin Life, 2024

Copyright © Billy Garvey, 2024

The moral right of the author has been asserted.

All rights reserved. No part of this publication may be reproduced, published, performed in public or communicated to the public in any form or by any means without prior written permission from Penguin Random House Australia Pty Ltd or its authorised licensees.

Cover design by Christa Moffitt, Christabella Designs © Penguin Random House Australia Pty Ltd
Volcano image by RN 3540/Shutterstock
Author photograph by Meagan Harding
Typeset in 12/18pt ITC Berkleley Old Style by Midland Typesetters, Australia

Printed and bound in Australia by Griffin Press, an accredited ISO AS/NZS 14001 Environmental Management Systems printer

NATIONAL LIBRARY OF AUSTRALIA
A catalogue record for this book is available from the National Library of Australia

ISBN 978 1 76134 583 8

penguin.com.au

FSC www.fsc.org MIX Paper | Supporting responsible forestry FSC® C018684

We at Penguin Random House Australia acknowledge that Aboriginal and Torres Strait Islander peoples are the Traditional Custodians and the first storytellers of the lands on which we live and work. We honour Aboriginal and Torres Strait Islander peoples' continuous connection to Country, waters, skies and communities. We celebrate Aboriginal and Torres Strait Islander stories, traditions and living cultures; and we pay our respects to Elders past and present.

This book is for my children, Yvette and Charlie. I haven't written it to help their mental health – I hope to do that in person in the years ahead – but to help their peers'. The generation coming up through childhood now will be my children's community, and I hope that in some small way I've made it a kinder place for them and those they share it with.

Contents

Introduction

The one universal truth of childhood is that there is always hope. As a developmental paediatrician who has worked with families for over twenty years, I've seen the most unsettled babies learn to be soothed, the wildest toddlers have their energy steered towards desired behaviours, the most sensitive kids thrive emotionally and the 'baddest' teens find themselves.

My clinical practice ranges from helping babies in their first weeks of life who are finding the cold and hungry outside world a little tough, to working with teens on the brink of adulthood who are battling mental illness that overwhelms them and their loved ones. This book aims to help you support children at any stage in that journey. If you're caring for a young child, this book is for you. If you're parenting a teenager, this book is also for you. My aim is to help you build the required skills to help children and teenagers by explaining the key developmental stages our kids go through, as they relate to mental health. So often we assume that time on its own will teach our children these important skills. But time teaches us nothing. Just because a child can fall asleep on their own doesn't mean they've learnt how to self-soothe. A child in primary school may still struggle with tantrums, and a teenager may have missed crucial aspects of attachment. All children are at risk of people seeing their age, not the specific thing they need help with. When we expect our kids to have figured things out simply because they're a certain age, we can set them up to fail. One of the best things we can do instead is to first lower our expectations, meet children at their current level of functioning and gently help them to further develop their skills in the particular area they are struggling with.

In these pages I will share what I've learnt about fostering strong mental wellbeing in children to give them the best chance of avoiding future mental illness. Fourteen years of study at university has provided me with a scientific lens to help, but it's the honesty and trust of the people I've met in the clinic that have given me an insight into the biggest challenges, fears and regrets our kids experience. I've learnt from each and every person, and I thank them. Research has guided my approach, of course, but it's children who have taught me what works. Please note that while I have changed names and personal details of the individuals I write about in this book to protect their privacy, the underlying stories are real.

Many of us feel lost as parents, wishing there was a guidebook to help navigate the rugged terrain of raising our children to be happy, healthy individuals. This book is aimed at developing our skills as parents and guardians to better face whatever challenges we find in the journey ahead. We will also explore how to respond to our kids' emotions, including when these emotions have deteriorated into mental illness. While I can't see each reader personally, I hope to share some of what you might experience when seeing someone like me in a clinic. It is becoming increasingly difficult to access specialist support as waitlists all around the world increase due to more children struggling and services being under-resourced. This harsh reality further burdens those desperate to find help and often worsens the challenges faced by the children we care for. Identifying and addressing mental health difficulties as soon as possible is the best chance we have of them improving, yet so many families are waiting years to see an experienced professional. Most are never seen. There is hope though. I'm here to tell you that there is no magic behind those closed doors and life does not happen in a consulting room. The children I meet in my clinic still require guidance in the real world. If you're unable to access professional support right now, don't be disheartened. There is still a lot you can do to guide and support your child as they face life's challenges.

I hope this book provides clear and achievable pathways through some of these challenges. Regardless of your child's age, I would encourage you to read this book from beginning to end so that you understand each stage of development. If you have a young child, it will set them up for their future. If you have a teen, it is not too late to go back and focus on the core issues of development and wellbeing.

Our society is drowning in mental anguish, and so much of the burden in our daily lives seems to be a fate we must accept. Suicide is one of the leading causes of death for teenagers and our adult peers.[1] It devastates families and broader communities in a way that few other fatal illnesses do. I believe this is because such shattering loss is actually preventable, and this knowledge compounds such needless suffering.

Adult mental health services worldwide tend to be reserved for those with resources or severe and chronic illness. But the majority of adult mental illness begins in childhood, usually before the teenage years.[2] Without appropriate support, the adversity of these early stages of mental illness can have lifelong consequences for an individual's self-esteem, relationships and daily functioning.[3] But no child, regardless of their environment or temperament, is destined to experience mental illness.

When I meet a child in the clinic I always wish I had helped them much sooner in their struggle. For anyone out there feeling like the children they support are struggling more than you can handle, please seek help. At the first sign of an issue, I would urge you to make an appointment with your family general practitioner or, for younger children yet to start school, with your maternal child health nurse. While you are waiting to see a clinical specialist, there is much you can do to help any child who is struggling, so that by the time you get to that appointment things are actually better, not worse, or you might not even need the appointment anymore.

We must all have a good understanding of the early signs that a child is struggling, to ensure that we see these as soon as possible, rather than waiting for them to be completely overwhelmed before we do anything. This is doubly important because getting in to see a specialist is really difficult. The public system is so overwhelmed that many families wait years for their first appointment, which means that by the time a child with a mental illness sees a specialist like me, their condition has usually worsened to such a degree that the child, their family and the professionals who support them are exhausted and at a loss as to what to do. And it's no better for my colleagues working privately. The demand has got so high that for the first time, many of them are closing their books to new referrals.[4]

In the chapters ahead we will explore how to best equip our children with the skills they need for good mental health, and our role in responding to challenges when they arise. Our communities will be stronger if we can find a way to ensure that all of us are safe, valued and feel a sense of self-worth. Decades of science and studies illuminate the way. The trick is to find the sweet spot between the textbooks and real life.

In 2019 I applied for a Churchill Fellowship to explore how to better support parents in guiding their children's development and mental health. I still remember the final interview. As I was waiting nervously to be called for the last hurdle of a long application process, I found myself questioning my legitimacy to even be standing in this fancy building, wearing a suit I've never felt comfortable in. As I sat down in front of a panel of twelve interviewers, it took everything in me to remain composed. A well-dressed man in the middle of the group abruptly asked the first question: 'We've read your application and, frankly, I don't believe there is any evidence that how we raise our children impacts their mental health. Please explain yourself.' This book is an extended version of my answer to that question. Given that I was awarded the scholarship, I assume they found the answer I gave helpful. I hope you do too.

1. Attachment is where your child's mental health starts.

Chapter 1

Attachment

I'll never forget the humbling experience of the first night my daughter Yvette spent at home after her birth. I'd had a chance to hold her and interact with her for the first few days, which was wonderful, but I was so excited for her to be at home with us and to really begin the journey of raising this little being.

My partner, Annaliese, was pretty exhausted. She'd worked right up until the birth, caring for other pregnant women in her role as an obstetrics doctor, and probably didn't get much rest before Yvette was born. This was my time to shine, though. I was a leading expert in babies. I supervised the Unsettled Babies clinic in the biggest paediatric hospital in the country. I was a published researcher in unsettled babies, and I'd helped write the national guidelines that other clinicians use all around the world when they meet unsettled babies in their practice. I can still remember my confidence that evening, telling Annaliese to go to bed and get some rest. 'I've got this,' I reassured her.

I did not have it. I tried all the moves I'd been teaching people for over a decade, trying equally hard to settle Yvette and not wake Annaliese from her first proper sleep in days. After about two hours of crying, Annaliese came out, took Yvette, wrapped her inside her dressing gown and smiled at me. Yvette settled down almost instantly. In hindsight it's a beautiful memory, but at the time it was a really important lesson in understanding the difference between being an expert and real life.

We've known about attachment theory since the 1960s.[1] Prior to this, some 'experts' saw babies as blank slates, even prescribing a certain amount of crying as exercise for newborns.[2] Now we know that babies are born seeking attachment.[3] Forming a bond with their primary caregivers has been an evolutionary necessity for a helpless newborn to ensure that caregivers sacrifice resources for them. This is not the only purpose of the biological drive to connect, though. It also begins the lifelong journey of a child's social and emotional development. Most of what we learn about the world comes from our interaction with others. From birth, infants preference faces over other visual objects[4] and turn to familiar voices more than those of a stranger[5]. A baby's primary caregivers are the first of many other relationships, and so the foundation we build for them through attachment will stay with them throughout their entire life, long after we've gone.

I found it really hard to connect with Yvette for the first few months of her life. I was surrounded by messages telling me that the moment our children are born we instantly fall in love with them. Social media amplifies the life-changing experience that happens when you first lock eyes with your newborn baby. It's filled with parents telling us they've finally found their purpose, or talking about how it all came to them so naturally. I didn't experience that. I've held hundreds of newborn babies in my career, and I had to admit this didn't feel very different. I knew the practical stuff, like how to hold her and change her nappy, but that was about it. I had no idea how to connect with her or settle her. Fortunately, unlike some people in this situation, I knew I wasn't alone and that, despite what social media tells us, many parents feel lost in the beginning, and around 20 per cent of mothers experience antenatal or postnatal depression, which can add to this feeling.[6]

In the Unsettled Babies clinic, we meet families every week who are worried something is wrong, often because their baby is really unsettled – hence the name! – or because their baby isn't interacting with them as much as they expected. Parents might be worried there is an underlying reason for this, such as a hearing problem or a diagnosis like autism. Sometimes I discover in parents an underlying fear that all will be revealed and they're not good parents. It's a huge privilege to come into the lives of families at this point, and I still think regularly about many of them: their fear and desperation at the first appointment, and their pride and confidence at their last.

Six-week-old Amelia was one of the unsettled babies I met. She was the second child of mum Samantha and father Michael, who also had a two-year-old daughter, Lilly. It's a common misconception that it's only first-time parents who struggle. While many parents learn a great deal about parenting through their first child, temperamental differences in babies mean that there can be significant differences between siblings in the first few months of life.

A child's temperament is really a gauge of how they respond to their environment. Studies have shown that while temperament is fairly fixed from an early age, understanding temperament can help guide us in supporting individual children.[7]

Researchers have found that the majority of children have a fairly easy temperament.[8] They are flexible to new environments and experiences, predictable in their emotions and easily soothed. Lilly was in this group: she had always slept really well, fed perfectly and didn't take long to settle when she was upset. My son, Charlie, is like this too. In all the babies I've spent time with, I've never met a happier or calmer child. He is almost always settled and smiling, and on the rare occasions he cries it takes little effort to settle him. He makes Annaliese and I look like superparents, when in reality it is just his easy-going nature shining through.

There's a second, smaller group of children who can be hesitant or take time to be comfortable in new environments or experiences but will generally get to a point of comfort and predictability with time. Yvette falls into this group. It can take her a little while to relax when we go somewhere we haven't been before, or to be comfortable with a new person, but once she is settled, she usually remains that way in that place or with that person.

Amelia was in a third group of children, however. This group – a relatively small percentage of children – are consistently sensitive to their environment. Many of the children we meet in the clinic have sensitive temperaments. They are quick to react to their surroundings, particularly if change occurs. They often struggle with self-regulation and have a low tolerance of stress. They are sensitive to fear and can easily become upset. They will be vulnerable to big emotional responses, especially in unfamiliar environments or new experiences, and they can be difficult to predict. Sensitive kids thrive, however, when we understand how to best support them. A whole chapter of this book is dedicated to just how we do this (Chapter 4). A big mistake is thinking that children with emotional difficulties are struggling because we are failing as parents. In truth we are still learning how to meet their emotional needs in those tough moments. For babies, especially, it takes time to learn what works, since they can't tell us with words!

Within the first week of Amelia being born, Samantha knew something was different. She didn't feel the same connection to Amelia that she had with Lilly when she was a newborn. Soon after, she noticed that Amelia would often turn away from her, unresponsive to her settling techniques. She was also struggling with feeding. Samantha found Amelia to always be hungry but she would stop feeding within the first few minutes, distraught and inconsolable almost every time. Samantha and Michael were at a loss. They had no family around to help, and Michael was back working long hours after a short period of parental leave. Samantha was drowning at home juggling Lilly and Amelia, and told me that she wasn't sure how much longer she could take this pressure.

Amelia is one of the many babies who has taught me the reality of attachment theory. Some babies, like mine, come into the world instantly seeking connection and making us look like instant experts. Once we realised she was allergic to dairy, her easygoing temperament shone through. We learnt her preferences for settling, how she would show us she was enjoying something and early signs that she wasn't. After that first night at home when I had trouble getting her to settle, her temperament quickly made me feel like I was an expert again. Not all babies are like this though.

Amelia falls into a group of around 30 per cent of babies who will be significantly unsettled in the first few months of life.[9] You might be wondering what 'significantly unsettled' means. It used to be determined by how much a baby was crying, and only 'high criers' were considered at risk enough to receive support. A 'high crier' was a baby who cried for more than three hours a day, for more than three days per week, for at least three weeks. But what if they cried for two and a half hours on one of those three days? Did that mean 'Oh well, we won't help you'? Thankfully, we've changed how we define unsettled babies and now the level of parental concern is what guides us – as it should with everything.

A thorough assessment revealed that Amelia was thriving in her growth and development. She was putting on weight and advancing in her abilities as we would expect for a baby in their first few months. There were no red flags that prompted investigations such as blood tests or a trial of prescription formula. Every child we meet in the clinic requires a detailed history and examination as a core aspect of the care we provide. Amelia revealed no concerns in this regard, but underlying pathology – meaning an organic medical cause – exists in about 5 per cent of babies who are unsettled.[10] Conditions such as cow's milk protein intolerance are relatively rare, but they require specific treatment, so as a first step we must always consider these as a possible cause.

Now was the fun part. Her parents and I would learn together how to connect with Amelia. In the first three years of life, our brains go through a huge growth period. Like with a garden in springtime, we not only get to watch this beautiful period of flourishing take place, but we get involved, get our hands dirty and become a part of this flourishing process. In the first few years of life, our growing brains send out neural pathways, like growing vines, in a stage of proliferation. Stimulus such as sounds, touch, sights and smells guide these growing pathways. The same stimulus, or lack of it, dictates what is prioritised and what is pruned. This early phase of brain growth is a critical time to enrich an infant's environment and set them up for strong and healthy brain development. Like gardening, the trick is in knowing how to do this well.

Amelia was a unique infant, and there will never be another Amelia. There are, however, some universal truths about babies. Attachment theory tells us that there are three stages of attachment seeking in infants.[11]

The first is communicating the desire for connection. Babies do this mainly through crying. It's their first and most powerful form of language and it's critical that we reinforce it. Concerns that always responding to crying will negatively reinforce this behaviour are misplaced, especially in the first six months of a child's life. It is really important that babies learn early on that their distress will be responded to with comfort and care. This promotes healthy secure attachment, which is a key ingredient for their self-esteem and confidence in exploring the world.[12]

We also know that up until at least six to nine months of age, babies don't understand that people exist even though they can't see them.[13] You can test this theory by playing with your child using their favourite toy. When they are following and engaged with the toy, drop it out of their view (such as over the side of their highchair). Most babies younger than six months of age won't look around for the toy as they think because they can't see it, it must not exist anymore. Understanding that a toy, or parent, exists even though you can't see it is called 'object permanence'. Even in children who have developed this skill, it is important that we show them we will come to them for comfort when they are distressed. For children who haven't yet learnt object permanence, it is really important that we understand the vulnerability in leaving them alone to cry out their distress. They don't know we are just in the next room, and so they might feel like their efforts to seek support are useless, meaning they are not developing that essential healthy attachment to their caregivers that is so important to their mental health later in life.

From around six weeks of age, babies learn more complex ways to reinforce this connection. The first true smiles from a baby are some of the most phenomenal experiences a parent can have. A smile lights up our own brain circuitry in a way that promotes attachment in us.[14] Another important lesson exists in this experience: attachment goes both ways. These interactions teach us how to best interact with and respond to the needs of our babies. Like any skill development as an adult, it can be a slow process, but it will benefit from repetition and realistic expectations. Soon after smiles come cooing, giggling and calling out, and these too are important skills to reinforce through your response and imitation (see breakout box).

Crying will dominate their repertoire, though, and it's crucial that we understand the importance of this.

Other types of feedback are critical to be aware of too. Infants will often hold your gaze when they are enjoying something, a great opportunity to return this and show our delight in them through smiling, talking and other expressions of joy such as laughter and singing. Equally, they will often turn away when they are overstimulated. These signs, along with tensing up and back arching, can be early ways that they guide us in what is helping them and what is not.

The second stage of attachment seeking – and the one we're trying to avoid – is giving up. When an infant learns that crying does *not* result in someone helping them, they will stop crying. This is different to an infant settling through comforting and soothing. It's also the reason that we need to keep comforting an infant even if they are still crying while we do it. Too many parents feel like their attempts are failing because their baby continues to cry. Like older children and adults, infants often struggle to regulate their emotions, despite our best efforts to soothe them, but this doesn't mean our efforts are wasted – far from it. While the infant is in distress, our support shows them that seeking help works, and that we are there for them. It doesn't mean our comforting isn't working. This is one of the most important lessons in this chapter. Our support should not be conditional on it resolving their distress.

The third stage – the one we don't want to get to – is a loss of attachment. After repeated and prolonged periods of unmet crying, a baby will learn the lesson that help doesn't come when they are distressed. Please don't misunderstand: loss of attachment doesn't happen with a baby who is occasionally left to cry while a parent takes a moment for themselves – or even goes and screams into a pillow! Moves like that are crucial to safely surviving the first few months of an unsettled baby's journey. Ensuring that parents put their babies down safely and walk away when they need to from time to time is a critical part of our clinical work.

A true loss of attachment happens after consistent, sustained and repeated periods of a child being left alone, and it is one of the most dangerous experiences an infant can have. Orphanages in eastern Europe played this out in real life. Babies were kept warm and fed but they were rarely held and soothed. The rates of mental illness in these children skyrocketed despite their basic needs being met.[15]

With Amelia, we knew that she was communicating her need for support and her parents were responding to this communication. She was still in the first stage of attachment-seeking, so we needed to figure out what moves helped her to settle when she was distressed. Each baby is different, so when we are learning what works for them, it's really important that we give specific approaches time to take effect. Often, desperate caregivers will shuffle between strategies really quickly, going from rocking, to patting, to feeding, to pacifying all within a matter of minutes. If we put ourselves in the position of these babies, we can start to imagine how unhelpful that might be. While well intended, rapidly shifting from one approach to another does little to provide a sense of calm.

The first step of working out what will settle your child is to pick a soothing method and give it a chance to work by doing it consistently for at least five minutes. How do you pick the method? Most methods are built upon an attempt to replicate life in the womb. Warmth and a tight wrap simulate the feel of this early environment, while rhythmic patting, walking and shushing replicate the sensation and sound of the mother's heartbeat. The womb is where babies first learn safety, so taking them back there is a really nice approach to comforting them.

The second, and most important step, is trying to be calm ourselves. Ideally we are calm when trying to calm a baby, as co-regulation is a really important aspect of mental health first aid (more on this in Chapter 2). In reality, this often feels impossible, but it's really important that we still try, using methods such as taking deep, slow breaths and slowing our own movements, or making them rhythmic. Babies will pick up on these attempts and learn early aspects of their own self-regulation. Thankfully, even if we don't always achieve the perfect calm state instantly, our babies get to experience the most important part of self-regulation: learning how to do it together.

Face stories

One of the most helpful techniques I use to coregulate and connect with Yvette is not something I learnt from a textbook or another clinical specialist, but from my mum. When I was little, she used to tell me face stories to strengthen our bond and calm both of us down when I was distressed.

I've taught Annaliese face stories too and we both use them with Yvette, who frequently asks for them, to my absolute delight, even occasionally when she is upset. She lies down and closes her eyes, and I gently place my index finger somewhere on her face, for example, behind one ear, and I start telling a story. It could be anything: 'One morning a cranky bear woke up from his nap. He gave a big stretch and yawn and went exploring,' I say, and start to softly trace my finger across her face. 'First he had a drink from a nearby pool because he was thirsty.' I carefully touch her closed eyelid. '"That feels better," he said. "Now I think I'll go find some berries in the forest."' I continue to trace my finger around her face as I tell the rest of the story for a few minutes, and then I gently tickle her nose to get her to open her eyes.

In these moments, Yvette and I are totally connected to each other. Usually it is just a nice activity to do after more active play or in place of a bedtime book when I want her to settle down. This helps to build our skills in coregulation so that we can call upon it during times of difficulty. I hope Yvette and Charlie pass this down to their kids one day too.

Engaging with an infant

We often think of crying as the only way babies communicate their desire to connect, but from only a few weeks of age, they have *many* skills in seeking connection or showing that they are enjoying or not enjoying an experience. Babies often reinforce a connection by holding our gaze, moving their limbs towards us, relaxing their bodies and seeking physical connection through touch. Equally, looking or moving away, tensing up or lashing out might be signs they are not enjoying an experience.

All are important opportunities for caregivers to respond, and they teach us how each individual baby communicates their feelings and needs. While we don't need to respond to *all* of an infant's attempts to communicate, it is important that we do respond often and are as present as possible when we do.

There are two key ways that we can engage: imitation and soothing.

Imitation teaches early social skills to babies, and it is a beautiful way to playfully support their development. Matching facial expressions, body movements and sounds helps them learn that we are similar to them and have feelings that we communicate too. These experiences bring joy, which helps us to form a secure bond with the infant in return. This form of interaction sets up future ways that the infant will connect with others. If we observe differences in this matching and the exchange is not successful, it can be a sign that the connection isn't working.

When babies communicate through crying, it is important that we soothe them, showing them their message of distress is being received. Some will like physical soothing that replicates the womb, such as tight wraps and heavy pacing around a room. Others will prefer a soft rhythmic voice repeating a sound or song. Most of what works is repetitive and soothing in a way that calms our own nervous systems, too. We should always remember our goal is not necessarily to stop the crying, but to see the act of soothing as an opportunity to further build secure attachment through connection.

Engaging with an older child

Significant and ongoing emotional difficulties, such as being reactive, withdrawing or struggling to benefit from the help of others, can be a sign that an older child hasn't yet established secure attachment. If this is occurring, it is worth revisiting the key aspects of attachment.

Just like with babies, we need to put time into establishing secure attachment during times of calm when our brains are most capable of forming new connections. The same principles that we use with babies apply to older children and teenagers too. Being present, emotionally available, responding to their signals consistently and providing comfort and protection all help to form bonds that will in turn help to build strong and secure attachment.

As the three stages of attachment seeking show, many babies who experience difficulties in settling risk missing out on developing a secure attachment with their primary caregivers, because they're not receiving the response they need to their distress, even if their parent is trying their best!

In my clinic, I ask all families what the first year (or weeks or months, if that's the case) has been like supporting their child, even when the children I'm meeting are in their late teens. Often when we explore this early period we find clues to the difficulties the child is having now. Difficult pregnancies, traumatic births, relationship strains and sleepless nights are common stories that shatter the fairytale of having a new baby. If a baby is still unsettled towards the end of their first year of life, they are ten times more likely to have developmental concerns at school entry.[16]

Why would I bring up these experiences in older children, though, if the crucial window of attachment has passed? Because it hasn't. Children who missed out on establishing secure attachment are not doomed to difficult lives, poor relationships and mental illness. Once we've identified the contributing factors, we can use the same principles that we do for babies to repair this insecure bond.

Older children and teenagers who missed healthy attachment in infancy first need to be shown they are safe and secure through responsive and predictable caregiving. Often we make the mistake of aiming too high with these strategies, expecting that one conversation will convince them that they are safe and secure. Just like with newborns, so much of a successful approach lies in hearing the distress, staying with them through it and figuring out what we can do to help – and for more than a few minutes. And what we often find is that many of the things that soothed us as infants still soothe us now. Limited language, a calm tone of voice and comfort over explanation helps all of us, not just distressed babies.

Over a number of months, Amelia taught Samantha, Michael and me how she liked to be settled. She had the expected peak in crying at around twelve weeks of age but then turned a corner and spent more and more time awake and content. We found out that Amelia didn't like tight wraps, was pretty sensitive to noisy environments and preferred to be held by Samantha over anyone else. She loved skin to skin contact, being sung to and heavy-footed pacing around the living room. Understanding these preferences allowed Michael to gradually play a bigger role in her settling, and then others. Lilly was able to interact with her little sister more too, including singing her favourite nursery rhymes to her, and Samantha regained her confidence in juggling them both each day.

I can still remember saying goodbye to Samantha, Michael, Lilly and Amelia for the final time. For some reason they really made an impression on me. It might have been the experience of meeting this amazing mum who was honest enough to share her deepest fears. Samantha had been told by her own mother that she'd be a terrible parent, and so, when Amelia was so unsettled, she was worried that this proved her mother was right. Maybe it was how much I was able to learn from Amelia through the stories her parents told me about her home life and her time in my arms in the clinic. Or maybe it was the way her sister demonstrated her role by singing nursery rhymes for me in the clinic, grinning with pride as Amelia beamed smiles back at her older sister. Either way, Amelia and her family were a key part of my own learning in how to best support the unsettled babies we meet in our life, and how addressing attachment can redirect development and help everyone in a family thrive.

Key lessons from Chapter 1:

- Babies are born seeking attachment. This bond with their caregivers is essential to lay the foundation for their social and emotional development and mental health later in life.
- Attachment is two-way, and is formed through being present, engaging with your child, comforting them and helping them feel valued and safe.
- It's never too late to identify and work on issues with attachment. While so much of attachment research talks about the importance of the first year of life, we don't stop seeking attachment and connections with others once this period ends. You can repair lost connections by creating opportunities for positive and meaningful interactions that are solely to show interest, care and love.

Strategies for parents:

- Look at the individual child's preferences and reactions to learn how to soothe them when they are in distress, to help achieve a healthy attachment.
- Invest as much time and energy as you can into being 100 per cent present with your child for some time each day. This investment will pay off!
- Try a strategy for at least five minutes before deciding that it's not working. Children may take a while to notice or adapt to the new situation before responding.
- Keep comforting a child even if you feel like your attempts are not working. It is making a difference.

2. There is always a reason behind a child's behavioural difficulties.

Chapter 2

Behaviour

I'd heard a lot about Max long before I met him. First in casual conversations at work mentioning a child people were really worried about, then more formally in the case conferences I participate in, with professionals who are combining their powers to try to help kids who are really struggling. Max was a three-year-old boy with really challenging behaviours. He wasn't allowed to attend any of the local childcare centres anymore, due to his violent outbursts, and his mum was at tipping point despite the multiple services providing support every day.

Max desperately needed to learn how to handle his emotions, because he was missing out on too many healthy and rich experiences with his family members and other peers. If we didn't start building his skill set, Max would likely become one of the many children I see who are unable to attend school due to safety concerns.

I was told that Max would enter a room with his fists clenched, ready to strike out if anything set him off. It didn't take much for Max to explode, which meant that at home his mum, Crystal, and three older sisters would do everything they could to please him. When he was really upset, all it took was someone making a sound for him to lash out. Multiple times a day he would hit either Crystal or one of his sisters just for talking or making noise while moving around the house. Most of his interactions with others were like this, leading to significant family distress and isolation. His youngest sister was terrified of him and would do everything she could to leave a room whenever he entered. Crystal told me she would never speak when he was around, which gave me a really important goal to aim for that would signal we were on the right path: Max and his sister having positive and healthy interactions. Sibling relationships build our blueprint for future peer relationships, and both Max and his sister needed to learn how to interact safely and successfully.

Over the years as a developmental paediatrician, I've met lots of kids with behavioural difficulties, but it was during my six years working at a childcare centre when I left school that I spent the longest period of time with them. The childcare centre was in one of Melbourne's most disadvantaged communities, a centre I had attended myself, first as a preschooler and then as a schoolkid needing after-school care and vacation care. I'd hated the place as a kid. My mum worked next door as a community engagement officer for the local council, and I was usually angry at my mum that my little brother and I were left there for such long hours. While she had no other choice than to leave us there, I did have a choice about *working* there. I'm still surprised I applied for the job.

I learnt more in this role about child development and mental health than in all of my years of university study. Many experts of child development and mental health haven't spent much time around children in their normal daily lives. This is why the most important experts when it comes to individual children are their caregivers. No one can ever understand and advocate as well for a child as their parents. Second place goes to educators, who spend more time with children in a day than I will in a year of seeing them in the clinic. Most of my colleagues in childcare went on to become amazing educators in the community we grew up in, whereas my own experience showed me that I wasn't cut out for it. Thankfully, meeting with kids again in the clinic showed me I could help them in other ways.

Every Wednesday morning, in one of the biggest children's hospitals in the world, I work in the Behaviour Clinic. Here we see children who have waited a long time, often over two years, for assessment and treatment of their behavioural difficulties. Most of my colleagues think I'm crazy when I say it's my favourite clinic, but there are a few very valid reasons why. First, the potential success is so meaningful. Families come in with heartbreaking stories of constant distress and worries about the kids. They are at their limit mentally, often caring for children who can no longer attend school due to their behaviour. In the first appointment with a family I hear their story, often one in which they detail bad behaviour, household stress and not knowing what to do anymore. Helping to turn that experience around for both the child and their family, knowing we are making a difference to all of their futures, is one of the most rewarding experiences for those of us who work in this space.

Second, it's here that I get to play detective. The clues are in the child's behaviour, and my job is to find the underlying reason. And there is always a reason. Children with behavioural difficulties don't wake up in the morning plotting to make everyone's life difficult. Their behaviours are flares that they send up, signalling that something – or multiple things – is not working for them. When we start to see behaviour like this, rather than as an intentional effort to annoy us, we have a much greater chance of finding out what's going on below the surface.

Third, working in the Behaviour Clinic is a nice reminder of my role in guiding my children when they are sending up their own flares. Every day I go home to opportunities to practise what I preach. I fail frequently, but I can use these stories to show parents that even the so-called experts can't do this perfectly. Perfect isn't my aim, though – growth towards better is.

Behavioural difficulties are really common, especially in younger kids like Max. Tantrums first start to appear in the second year of life, when children develop skills that mean they can influence their environment, such as more mobility and speech. The challenge is that while they rapidly acquire these abilities, they are a long way off figuring out two other really important skills: emotional regulation and theory of mind. Theory of mind is understanding that other people have different experiences from our own. It is an essential piece of the puzzle of childhood development that many children with poor social skills have missed, and a topic we will discuss more in Chapter 7.

Anyone expecting very young kids to understand another person's perspective and feelings is setting themselves, and the child, up for failure. Instead, emotional regulation should always be the first step: a child must get to know their own feelings and how to react to them before they can learn about other people's. And as mentioned in Chapter 1, parents need to learn to regulate their emotions too. We often go straight to telling off kids because they've upset another child, or behaved in a way that shows they don't understand another person's feelings (including ours). But the issue with this is that at best a child won't understand what they've done wrong, and at worst it may set off their own emotional difficulties, further reinforcing the negative experience.

For example, when young children fight over a toy, we might make the mistake of scolding the child for snatching. What we can do instead is start by recognising the feeling the child has (excited to play with the toy and anger at not getting to) to validate them, then help them to understand the other child's feelings (happy to be playing with the toy and would be sad if it was taken). Then we can help guide them to the expected behaviour (playing with another toy until the child has finished with this one) and reinforce this sharing and patience through immediate and specific praise. This gives the child the best chance to feel validated in their own feelings, and provides an opportunity to learn about the other child's perspective and a healthy way to manage the situation.

To the relief of exhausted parents, most children's tantrums settle down by four to five years of age.[1] I do worry, however, that rather than truly learning to regulate their emotions, many children learn to either hide these feelings or avoid anything that might lead to similar unwanted feelings inside themselves. The negative consequences of displaying emotional difficulties, or not receiving the support they need, teach them that these are not safe feelings to communicate to others. This can echo through adult life, impacting an individual's self-esteem, relationships and mental health. Our expectations of how others will respond to our emotions is built in childhood, and it can be difficult to rebuild a sense that expressing feelings such as anger and sadness is okay if you've been shown the opposite. This can lead to social conflict and heightened anxiety if not addressed. This is why we can still use the following strategies to support older children and teenagers who have uncontrolled emotions, repressed feelings or avoidant behaviours.

Often in the clinic I find myself drawing. I'm not great at it, but it can be helpful for explaining certain concepts and to simplify complex theories. There is one illustration I do over and over again:

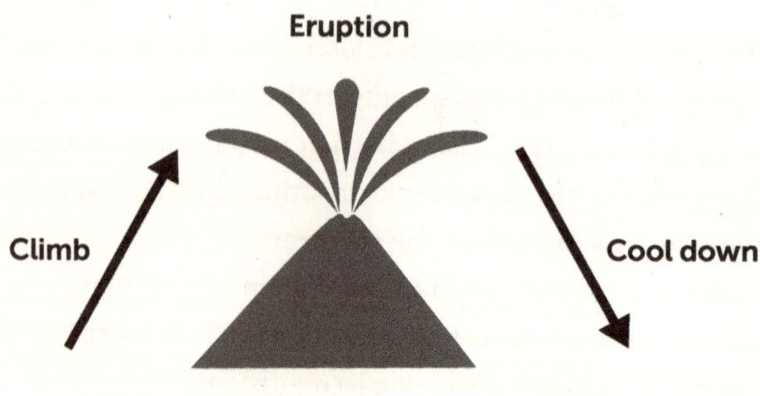

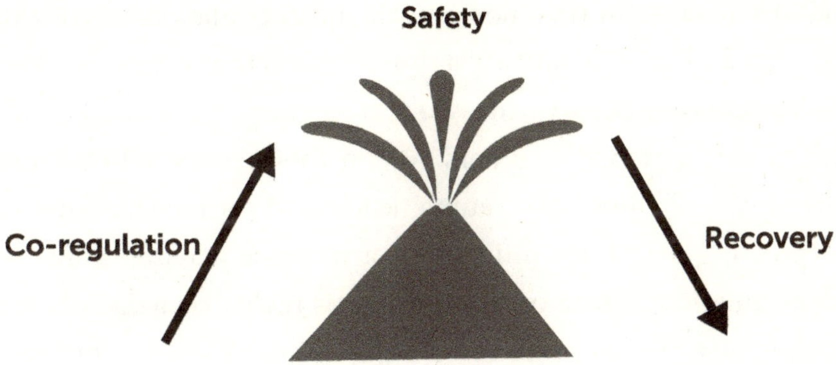

I like to think of kids with behavioural difficulties as volcanos. They don't have much control over when they erupt, and experts study them for early warning signs of a catastrophic explosion. Those early warning signs are what I look for, and what I try to teach families like Max's to spot. Not because we want to stop eruptions (I'm not sure if volcanoes feel relief after they blow, but I know that kids – and adults – can benefit from letting off steam) but because, as I'll explain later, it's an opportunity to guide their emotional regulation.

There are three parts to the volcano exploding. First is the climb, where pressure builds and rumbling tremors occur. The second stage is the fiery explosion. The third and final stage is the cool-down.

Most people want to know what to do during the explosion but the truth is, just like real volcanoes, safety is all that matters. Safety for those around the child, but most importantly, safety for the child too. Kids with behavioural difficulties, especially those with a history of trauma, benefit greatly from safety being the priority when they are dysregulated. If safety isn't prioritised in this moment, then dysregulation is likely to worsen for the child and all of those around them. This can lead to devastating consequences, such as property damage, self-harm and violence to others. When this occurs, all involved are at risk of emotional trauma, leading to future avoidance of expressing emotional difficulties or increased susceptibility to dysregulation. Educators deal with this reality on a daily basis, highlighting the need for better support and resources for these professionals.

After safety, the next thing to pay attention to are the signs building up to the eruption. All kids have different ways that they show a possible explosion. For my Yvette, it's erratic behaviour. When she's not getting what she wants, she will throw anything within reach across the room. Sometimes it's a spoon, at other times her favourite doll. Next, she will start throwing herself around. She runs, jumps, flails her arms and throws herself onto the floor. I often find myself smiling at this little person lying facedown with her ginger mop of hair splayed out, taking up almost as much floor space as her body. Her final signal is a verbal eruption. She screams at the top of her lungs as the built-up emotions escape her body. If I wait for her to start screaming, I know I've missed my chance before she erupts, and I go straight to safety. If I catch her earlier though, I have a chance to guide her emotional regulation. Let me walk you through how I do this.

Just yesterday I was sitting with her, playing Lego. She was building a fairly abstract airport and I was resisting every urge to follow the actual instructions. She couldn't get one of the pieces in and started hitting it against the others. Next, the piece went flying through the air. I had a split-second window where she looked at me, so I looked at her, picked up a different piece and threw it gently across the room, where it landed next to her piece. I then said, 'Silly Lego,' picked up another piece and threw that one too. We then both sat there and happily played a new game of throwing Lego across the room. After a short while, when I was sure she had returned to calm, we got the piece she was struggling with and tried again. What we'd just pulled off together is called co-regulation. Yvette started to become dysregulated, and I was able to remain calm, connect with her and then help her to return to feeling calm too. I didn't distract her or use lots of words, but instead I tried to help her understand her experience. In her mind the Lego was being silly, which is a valid feeling for a two-year-old.

Many of the coping mechanisms I use in my daughter's moments of frustration have the same strategy of finding an outlet for the difficult emotions, but I'd be lying if I said this works all the time. In the beginning, I pretty much always found I needed to be the person ensuring everyone was safe, as we couldn't stop the eruptions. With time, however, I started to learn Yvette's cues, feeling them in myself too, and experimented with strategies to help her return to a state of calm. We have to remember that children learn nothing in isolation. I can spend five hours a day in a room with a violin, but I'm not going to learn to play it if no one shows me how.

Finally, while it is important to pay attention to the cool-down, this isn't the priority. I often see well-intentioned families trying to do the work here. Parents will talk to kids after the event, trying to understand what happened, sometimes enforcing punishment in the hope that they will prevent future episodes. 'Why did you throw the Lego, Yvette? You should have asked for help. Next time we will have to stop playing if you do that.' We do the same with older kids. Sitting on the couch or the edge of their bed at the end of the day, talking about something that has gone wrong at home or school. There is nothing wrong with this approach, especially if the priority is to improve our understanding of the child's experience in order to be better equipped to help them next time. It's also a wonderful opportunity to show kids that we are unconditionally supportive and in partnership with them. We have to make sure we approach it with this goal, though, and not expect that a stern conversation will somehow mean they suddenly acquire the skills needed to navigate difficult feelings the next time they come up.

There is also risk in our help only being provided after the eruption. The first risk is that kids who send up these flares just want help. If the only time we give them this help is after the eruption, we may be unintentionally teaching them that this is the only way to get help. The kid in a classroom who explodes and gets sent to the principal's office cares more about ending the uncomfortable experience than not getting in trouble. They've learnt that when they are struggling, the flare of eruption works in terms of ending that experience. Showing them that support can come during or, ideally, *before* the eruption, helps them to feel safe and builds their skills in handling these tough feelings. The second risk is that just because a child can explain what happened after everything has settled, and maybe even promise it won't happen again, does not mean that they will manage things any differently the next time. Bright and articulate children are especially vulnerable to this second risk. Every week I meet frustrated parents who tell me, 'My child can tell me exactly what they did wrong and that they won't do it again, but it never gets better.' 'Getting better' at erupting is all about emotional regulation. Emotional regulation isn't learnt in the eruption or the cool-down though, it's learnt in the climb.

Regulation versus reflection

We've all blown up over something minor, such as being cut off in traffic, then thought later, 'That was a bit silly of me', once we've cooled down. It is almost impossible to remember that the next time you get cut off, though, isn't it? That's because these are two completely different skills. Realising you were silly after the event isn't emotional regulation, it's reflection. Reflection helps us to think about our role in scenarios after they have happened, but the real skill of emotional regulation is developed in the moment you get cut off, through awareness of your own feelings in that moment.

As we discussed in Chapter 1 about attachment, our brains are built for connection. This is the main reason we have succeeded as the dominant species on the planet. From the moment they enter the world, newborn babies seek out faces, voices and touch to help their brains wire neural connections. As children get older, they can play a more active role in seeking out and creating these rich experiences, which promote growth in the emotional and social parts of their brain. Kids who act out are seeking the same connection. Those who act out so much that it is negatively impacting their relationships often haven't figured out how to do it in a healthier way. They need support to learn how connection can help them to return to a state of calm, which is the basis of co-regulation. The first step in co-regulation is not actually connection, though, it's self-regulation. It's not for the child, but us.

Co-regulation is how we *learn* self-regulation, hopefully during childhood. Self-regulation is our ability to observe our own feelings and emotions and maintain control of our behavioural response. Before we attempt to connect with a dysregulated child, we must ensure that we have checked in with our own feelings and are calm. If we try to help a child return to calm but we ourselves are also dysregulated, what often happens is that we further dysregulate each other, an outcome none of us want!

We all have different skills at self-regulation, given how closely it is tied to our own temperament and our own upbringing. Annaliese finds it much easier to self-regulate than I do. This used to drive me crazy, until I realised that I just needed more practice for me to get to her skill level in calming myself during stressful parenting moments. Once I'd accepted that and given myself a fair chance to learn, it was much easier to achieve it. In the words of the amazing cartoon *Adventure Time*,

'The first step at being good at something is sucking at it.' Once we get good at it, we can then go to step two: co-regulation.

Connecting with kids who are in the pressure-building phase of the volcano can be tough, and once they have erupted we've lost any chance for the connection to form. They've lost access to the higher functioning parts of their brain that process information and apply reason, and their emotions trigger a flood of changes in blood flow, hormones and neural activation. Just like the scientists trying to predict the small seismic changes that come before the volcanic lava explosion, we too need to learn the early signs. I am constantly learning them from Yvette, as I discussed earlier with the Lego story, and in the clinic, I needed to help Max's mum learn them from him. When we register these signs and we have found our own calm, we can then try to engage with the child before they erupt.

Most of this connection is done non-verbally, through co-regulation. With young children, it's a good idea to get down to their level and keep our bodies relaxed, our breathing slow and our facial expression calm. By responding to their behaviours in this way, we are modelling regulation, and hoping they respond to our calm state by regulating their own system. This is called mirroring and our brains love to build neuron connections when it happens.

If we do speak, what we say is really important. Many of us use the phrase 'It's okay'. While seemingly harmless, this statement isn't great for two reasons. The first is that for the child, it *isn't* okay. As we will discuss in Chapter 4, all emotions are valid, it's the behaviour that follows them that we are trying to work on. For Yvette, it wasn't okay that the Lego didn't go where she wanted it to – it was a threat to her ability to master the perfect abstract airport she was trying to build. The second reason is that saying 'It's okay' also risks diminishing our own role in helping a child who is struggling. This is why I prefer 'I'm here'. It shows kids that we will be there for them whatever is happening, and it reminds us that our role is to help with those tricky feelings and not expect that they be pushed down to either later erupt or be hidden in future challenges.

While older kids may have moved on from throwing Lego, the same principle applies. We can help validate their experience by connecting over whatever frustration they are facing. It might be missing out on being picked for the netball team or a falling out with a friend that prompts us to guide them to express their emotions safely, through actions and language that works for them. 'I can see you're upset. I'd like to understand so I can help.' Saying this from a genuinely curious and supportive perspective, without judgement or frustration, shows our intention to support. Non-verbal components are integral here too. A calm tone of voice, relaxed posture and open body language gives us the best chance to guide the child or teen to be calm, too.

Back to Max, the three-year-old I met in the Behaviour Clinic. We knew from his body language, shouting and treatment of his siblings that he was consistently dysregulated and erupting in a way that was affecting him greatly, along with the rest of the family. Before we could even begin to understand the early signs for an eruption from Max, though, and teach Crystal to use co-regulation with him, we needed to help her with her own self-regulation.

Max's father was no longer on the scene, but he'd left a lasting impression. He was a huge, violent and explosive man who would enforce his rule over others through physical intimidation and violence. Learning this helped me to understand where Max had learnt this behaviour and also gave me an insight into why his mum and sisters were struggling so much when they saw this all over again from Max.

Despite being a tiny and angelic-looking boy, Max had learnt from his dad how to be in control. The first time I met him in the clinic, he walked up next to my chair, locked eyes with me and raised his clenched fist at my face. I had to practise what I preach and show Max I was calm and that he was safe. The world is a scary place for a three-year-old who feels he has complete control of it, and Crystal needed to regain that control to help Max feel safe again in the world. Parental mental health has its own chapter in this book (see Chapter 10), but Crystal is one of the many amazing parents who taught me its importance.

By prioritising Crystal, we made sure that Max had a secure and well-equipped primary caregiver to support him in any difficulties he faced. She was connected with a therapist who helped her process her own trauma. Services also provided practical support with finances and household logistics, such as school transport and food shopping, thereby reducing the stress she had to deal with to keep the family functioning. It was also essential that she was re-connected with her social group, a protective factor that had been intentionally removed from her life by her previous partner to increase his control over her. It took time, but it was wonderful to watch her stress reduce and her energy grow.

Once we'd learnt together how to build his mum's capacity, we then learnt the early signs of eruption for Max. He was almost the opposite of Yvette, because Max would shout and yell as his first sign of dysregulation, often at his sisters when he was not getting his way. Then his body would become tense, and he would tighten his little fists, squeezing and opening them repeatedly. His final stage was pounding whoever or whatever was in reach.

It took a long time for Max to learn how to co-regulate with his mum, but slowly and with lots of support she and then others were able to come in during the shouting phase to help him return to a state of calm. His hypersensitivity to everything around him and the consistent use of aggression as a response meant that we had to be gentle and patient to show him another way. It took consistency from all of those around him, ensuring they remained calm and in control, to signal that he was safe. By learning the early signs that Max was struggling – the shouting – his mum and others could work on signalling safety as soon as possible. Any shouting or yelling was met with a balance of soothing and control.

Crystal really struggled with this initially, but she found it easier after seeing the amazing early childhood educators demonstrate it at childcare. Max's hostility continued for a while, but the predictable response from others slowly calmed down his fear response and allowed him to be guided to more appropriate behaviours. First, he was guided to less destructive actions, such as jumping and slamming his body on mats (his bed at home) or tightly squeezing cushions. Then he slowly learnt words to match his emotions ('I'm angry'), followed by words to ask for support ('Please help'). These could then be reinforced and, over time, Max started to experience the positive benefits of interacting with others, and he could learn that these experiences were more rewarding than aggression and lashing out.

The child who taught me the most

I've spent countless hours researching, writing, reviewing and discussing the evidence about behavioural difficulties in children. Translating that research and theory into helpful and practical strategies has provided me with so many opportunities to help the families and professionals I meet in my clinical and education roles. As I've said, though, real life is always the best teacher and my biggest lesson came from one single interaction at childcare. I was running a school holiday program attended by sixty children that was the last chance for many children who were not allowed to attend other centres due to behavioural difficulties. An eleven-year-old boy named Jake had been sent to our centre after repeated acts of violence at others. I was busy when he arrived, but within minutes a commotion kicked up that alerted me he was here. I'd worked hard over many weeks to settle some of the aggressive kids at our centre, and on this occasion I became pretty dysregulated myself when I rushed over to see three of them fighting with a new boy who I guessed was Jake. Once the fight was broken up, Jake fled from the centre over one of the fences with me following close behind. I was about twenty years old at this stage, so my main response was to enforce my authority. My attempts failed, with Jake swearing at me and threatening me, further provoking me to enforce my role as the adult. Both of us were triggering the other into more elevated negative feelings. As the adult I should have known better, but in reality, I wasn't far from still being a kid myself.

Jake was in residential care, having been removed from his parents years ago. When he refused to return to within the safe boundary of the program, I called his caseworker to come and pick him up, showing him that I didn't need to tolerate his behaviour. Every day for that first week Jake demonstrated consistent behaviour of aggression, followed by escalation and then threats, and every day I sent him home early. One morning, though, I tried a different approach in an attempt to get ahead of a repeat of this pattern. I asked Jake to come and help me set up the obstacle course of the day. It got him out of the morning meeting, so he reluctantly came along with me. At the playground, I showed him how we should run the course. 'You start here on the balance beam, then onto the monkey bars, over the tyres, then the bridge, up the ladder and then down the slide. If you fall off anywhere, you get five seconds added to your time.'

I'd run it like this for years and it always seemed to work well.

'That's wrong,' Jake said. 'You should take time off for each bit they *don't* mess up instead of punishing them for falling. You're just focusing on the bits they stuff up.'

I couldn't believe it. An eleven-year-old who'd had a pretty terrible life so far could see that kids will do better and enjoy something more if you reinforce the good behaviours instead of punishing the bad ones. Decades of research have gone into that single concept, and I was taught it by a kid who'd probably never experienced it.

That following week with Jake was one of the most humbling experiences of my career, as now I saw that he was someone I could learn from instead of teach. He still had lots of violent outbursts, but I saw that it was my role to learn what the triggers and early signs were, try to remain calm, connect with him and guide him towards less-destructive behaviour. I looked for positive things to give attention to and reinforce in all of his behaviours, and gradually over that six weeks we spent together he found his place in the centre and connected with other kids there. I never saw Jake again after that holiday period as he was moved to another residential facility, but every time I think about the power of positive reinforcement, I think of him and hope that others saw that they could learn from him too.

Now that we had helped remove the biggest obstacle to Max succeeding in his world, which was his lack of emotional regulation, we were able to address the other reasons behind his behavioural difficulties. Crystal was really overwhelmed, and she needed support, and therapy for what had occurred during her own childhood and her relationship with Max's abusive father. Once her capacity started to build, we worked on other contributing factors like Max's poor sleep, diet and exercise. He was getting so little sleep that it was no wonder he was so agitated. His diet was pretty limited and his weight so low that he was constantly running on empty. He also needed a physical outlet to safely move his body and gain a sense of mastery in something other than conflict.

With a combination of these underlying factors, time and his greater emotional capacity, Max was able to see new ways to interact with people. He started to see others as a source of safety and calm instead of threats to his control. Returning to childcare gave him the opportunity to see safety in other adults besides his mother, and then learn how to navigate peer interactions with support. Slowly he learnt how to share, communicate his feelings and signal his need for help in healthier ways than violence. The last time I ever saw Max, Crystal came into the room first, with a sense of calm over her that I'd never seen. She was finally sleeping, supported and hopeful. I asked where Max was, and she said he was coming. Sticking my head out the door, I saw Max happily running down the corridor with his little sister, both giggling as they raced through the door and into my room. I glanced over at Crystal, smiling, not sure if she was aware this was the moment I'd been aiming for all along.

Key lessons from Chapter 2:

- Behaviours are expressions of emotions. Children with frequent difficult behaviours are sending up flares to tell us that they need more help. Our role is to try to discover what help is needed.
- When a child is really acting out, the best thing to do is to provide safety and support. The real skill development happens when the child first starts expressing those challenging emotions. Learning those early signs helps us to help kids before the challenging behaviour really kicks in.
- Often we make the mistake of trying to stop a behaviour. Rather, we should think about what we would like the child to do instead. If this is possible, then we give the amount of support required to help them carry out that expected behaviour and then reinforce it. The two biggest mistakes we make with guiding children to better behaviours is that the stretch is too much or we are not giving enough support.

Strategies for parents:

- No child or teenager intentionally makes life difficult with challenging behaviours. Outbursts and aggression are flares that they send up to show that they are struggling and want support or want a situation to end.
- The first step starts with us. As adults we must ensure that we are calm ourselves before we expect a child to find a state of calm. If we don't do this, we may actually make things worse, cause further escalation of behaviours or, even worse, cause the child to hide their difficult feelings altogether.
- When we have calmed ourselves, our goal is to connect with the child to help them find calm too. In being aware of our own verbal and non-verbal expressions, we can observe the child to see if they are beginning to settle as a result of our actions. This skill is learnt in partnership over many repetitions.

3. Strong social skills ensure healthy and positive relationships throughout our entire life.

Chapter 3

Social skills

Sophie was a three-year-old whirlwind the first time she entered my consulting room. I can still remember her mother, Lucy, profusely apologising as Sophie stormed past me to the toys and started hurling them out of the box and across the room, searching for something she wanted to play with.

It's an experience that people like myself who are working in this space often have, and it's a wonderful opportunity to show parents right from the start that we are comfortable with kids being kids, that we don't take things too seriously and that we understand their position. I often look for a specific aspect of the child I've just met to praise, genuinely delighting in the opportunity to meet them. Sophie gave me lots to work with here. Her energy and ability to quickly check out all of the toys were pretty impressive. I also told her that she was really good at picking which toy to play with, as the green truck with only one wheel was my favourite too. There is little use in having technical expertise if you can't connect with the people who it might help. It's my favourite part about my work, and I'm always trying to get better at it. Sophie also needed help to get better at making connections – that's why she and her mum were here.

Lucy described Sophie as a very boisterous happy girl, but she was really struggling socially. Sophie was the first child of Lucy and her partner, Sam, and they loved how much energy she had and that she showed no fear. Unfortunately, these same amazing qualities meant she really struggled with other kids her age. When Sophie turned two, Lucy returned to work but it didn't last long. Frequent stories of Sophie struggling in social interactions at childcare meant that Lucy had to pick her up early, then send her less often and then not at all. It was usually the same story: Sophie would rush in, grab toys from other kids, play rough and start to yell when she didn't get her way. This wasn't a problem at home as she was either playing on her own or with the responsive help of Lucy and Sam. They did notice this same behaviour, however, when they went to visit friends with kids. Lucy told me that Sophie's behaviour was starting to impact their adult friendships and causing anxiety for her and Sam when Sophie was playing with other children.

Emotional and social development are often discussed as if they go hand in hand, but in reality they are two very separate areas in which children experience success and struggle. Along with emotional development, social skills are the biggest predictor of lifelong success in terms of physical health, mental health, self-esteem and relationships.[1] As we will explore, emotional development is an internal process that both influences and is influenced by our interactions with others. Social development is all about those interactions. While there is a genetic influence on how quickly and easily children will acquire social skills, we as parents can have a huge impact on how adept our children become at navigating social situations.

At our core we are social beings. Our success – and survival – as a species has been earned over thousands of years of collective hardship and victory, and this has led to our brains being uniquely wired for independent thought but collective problem solving. While we are intelligent, it is our social abilities that make us truly unique. It feels good when we connect with someone, just as it crushes us when we are rejected. Our skills in making connections are honed over millions of social interactions, but the way we see, understand and navigate the social world is formed in childhood, beginning from our first days as an infant. The word 'infant' itself shows the history of misunderstanding of babies in this regard. In Latin it means 'without speech' and 'foolish'. We now know that the opposite of both descriptions is true. Infants are learning the moment they enter the world, including social behaviours from a very early age, as American psychologist Andrew Meltzoff demonstrated using copying behaviours.[2]

At the time of writing, my son, Charlie, is four months old. He is learning the basic steps for both verbal and non-verbal communication. Soon after birth, if I poked my tongue out, he would do the same thing back to me, beginning to realise that he and I are similar. This early imitation will become a pillar of all of Charlie's cognitive development throughout his life, as being able to see similarities in others is a key social skill. Some of our greatest delights and pangs of regret come from seeing our kids imitate what we've modelled to them, often unknowingly. (I'll never stop laughing at little Yvette imitating Annaliese as we pulled back out of the driveway a second time after forgetting something, chirpily stating, 'Let's try again.')

Now, at four months, Charlie is practising his verbal social skills, making babbling sounds to try to connect with me and his other family members. To help him develop these, I make sure I face him and try hard to imitate the sounds he makes. The closer I get to his babbling sounds, the more likely he is to continue the conversation. His smile when I really get it lights us both up. This successful exchange leads to a release of chemical neurotransmitters in both of our brains, which makes us feel good and therefore more likely to do it again.[3] This means I am helping him develop more complex abilities and we are deepening our connection.

While these exchanges are rich opportunities for attachment (see Chapter 1), they also help Charlie to learn the back and forth process of social interactions that he will need to succeed with the thousands of people he will meet during his life. The connection we build with our kids is their blueprint for future relationships. Through our social interactions with them, we can help them learn how to give and expect kindness, comfort, respect and gratitude in their relationships with others. These are known as prosocial skills, and how well our kids pick up on these will have a huge influence on their success in social settings such as early childcare, school and beyond.[4]

While Charlie can watch my tongue poke out and do the same with his, he can't yet understand that I'm a person with feelings (as discussed in relation to 'theory of mind' in

Chapter 1). Developing prosocial skills guides us towards understanding the feelings and needs of others, but many kids I meet in the clinic – including teenagers approaching adulthood – have missed essential steps in this journey and have not yet experienced true friendship as a result.

One key prosocial skill, which takes years to develop, is empathy. Empathy at its core is about connection, and it can help kids move away from the egocentricity of early childhood and develop kindness towards others. When we see someone suffering, empathy leads to the desire to help, which in turn builds our confidence and strengthens our self-esteem. It also has the benefit of bolstering the connection between the two individuals.

Like many skills, the development of empathy also starts in the first year of life. A baby often cries in response to another baby crying, which we know because there is no personal trigger, such as hunger, tiredness or a soiled nappy. This contagious aspect of emotions stays with us throughout our lives and is what helps us share our joy and suffering alike. After one year of age, a child's skills advance and they will often seek comfort themselves when someone else is distressed. The toddler that wants a hug when another child has been injured shows us this. The child has learnt that others can soothe their own distress, which is an essential aspect of development. In the early toddler years, however, they are yet to really understand distress in others or learn that in addition to receiving comfort, they can provide it too.

This is one of the reasons that neglect is so toxic to developing brains, because it means the child misses out on this essential life lesson. If comfort during distress never comes, that part of social development does not progress at all. When toddlers are comforted, though, they increasingly see the benefit of leaning into social connections in moments of difficulty.

The development of social skills really kicks up a notch in the toddler years. One of my favourite colleagues talks about how if toddlers were adults, many of them would be in jail. While those of us with toddlers can laugh at this, it also gives us an insight into one of the challenges of this period. The famous child psychologist Jean Piaget talked about this developmental period being one of 'egocentricity'.[5] To a two-year-old, the world is all about them. Usually after two years of age, children seek to soothe one another, but as they can only really see themselves in the world – they're not yet able to recognise other people's feelings – the soothing is only from this egocentric perspective.[6] For example, in an attempt to help, they will give the person who needs soothing their favourite toy or perform a soothing act they like such as cuddling or patting. This shows us that they don't yet understand that the needs of the other person may be different to their own. This understanding comes later, from around four years of age, and is mainly built during cooperative play and sharing.

My daughter, Yvette, two and a half at the time of writing, is further along this process than Charlie. As a toddler, she now has the communication and mobility skills needed to explore her world more broadly. Having a secure base to return to in Annaliese and me means she can confidently move away from us to test her skills with her peers and other adults. She often struggles socially; for example, being pushed out of the way on the slide or having a toy snatched from her grasp. By observing these interactions, however, I can see where her skills need more support. Yvette is on track for developing empathy and other prosocial skills, but she struggles to stick up for herself, finding it easier to let the kids on the slide push past her or to give up toys.

This is a common experience for girls in the playground, but that doesn't mean we can't work on it. In the safe environment of home, we help Yvette to understand and practise sticking up for herself using pretend play, modelling and stories. These play-based activities allow me to demonstrate how all of her toys should have a turn on the slide. We practise how a toy that misses out might respond, both the good and the bad. I mainly want her to know that she should expect things to be fair and how to speak up if she thinks they aren't, and then seek help from an adult if that doesn't work. As she gets more confident at these basic steps, I can guide her towards more advanced skills of sticking up for herself and conflict resolution. When we feel that she understands and can demonstrate this skill, we guide her in trying it out in more challenging environments like the playground. We closely watch to see how she goes and we increase our support if she struggles.

Competency in social skills is a key determinant of self-esteem and good mental health later in life.[7] In the clinic, I often meet older children who missed skill development in these early years or developed dysfunctional skills, meaning that they are stuck at a much earlier level of social development than other children their age. Adults think that because they are a certain age they should have figured it out by now, and so little or no support is provided. Our goal for all children in terms of social development should be that the majority of their social interactions are positive. For kids who do not have this experience, we have to find the specific reason why. In the clinic we often hear about how children play really well with older kids and younger kids but not those their own age. This is a common story for kids who are behind in their social development. The older kids will compensate for the child who is behind, so the play works okay, and the younger kids they play with are often at a similar level, meaning the play succeeds here too.

Other signs that a child is behind in their social development include unhealthy friendships, bullying and social isolation. Unhealthy friendships occur when children who have not developed prosocial skills, such as empathy, kindness and sharing, find each other. Because children are wired to build social connections, this can mean that they remain in unhealthy friendships where they are treated poorly by another. Relationships should elevate us, but by not expecting this from those we choose to spend time with, we can miss out on a very beneficial aspect of mental health. All three of these signs (unhealthy friendships, bullying and social isolation) can be signals of poor social skills and fragile self-esteem. This is true even for the child doing the bullying, as they use this behaviour to compensate for their inability to engage in positive social interactions. It's a way of protecting their self-esteem from fracturing as a result.

Many teenagers in our community have missed out on learning crucial social skills, and this can be hugely detrimental to their mental health and that of the people supporting them. Each week I meet teens who are socially isolated without a single good friend. I also meet teens in unhealthy social relationships, where unsafe risk-taking leads them down a path of potential harm to their future. Finding the social skills they are lacking and supporting them in developing these is just as important and achievable as it is with younger children. For example, if we do not support Yvette in establishing the ability to stick up for herself, she may go on to never learn that skill. This is likely to then lead to her really struggling with future conflict resolution, and she may fall into the pattern of always letting others have their way, or perhaps using aggressive tactics to resolve conflict. We all know adults like this, and we can see that they missed learning another way during their childhood.

Sophie wasn't showing signs of fragility in her self-esteem yet, but she was definitely at risk of it as she got older. She was missing opportunities to socialise with kids every day, because she was stuck at a much earlier stage of social development than her peers, and hadn't learnt yet how to successfully interact with others.

Clinical assessment is at the core of how developmental paediatricians learn how to help children like Sophie. Lucy explained that Sophie had had a strong and secure attachment early on, routinely being soothed during distress and showing confidence exploring the world as she became more mobile. She never really got too stressed, living proof that responsive and predictable early parenting can lessen stress reactivity in children.[8] She was, however, behind in her speech development.

Social skills require communication, just like dancing needs music. Communication is the foundation on which all social skills are built, and while not all communication is verbal, and many people learn to socialise without speech, for most of us it's a big part of the puzzle. At three years of age Sophie spoke only about twenty words, and she could follow a single-step instruction. This meant her speech development was below that of a typical two-year-old child. She also struggled to understand non-verbal body language. When I asked Lucy how Sophie would respond if Lucy was visibly upset, she said that Sophie wouldn't even notice.

Here we had found a key underlying reason for her difficulty succeeding with peers: Sophie was behind in her language development. There are several reasons this might have been the case, including language delay, poor hearing, intellectual disability and neurodiversity, including autism. Figuring out the skill gap and then addressing it is the key for so much of the work I do in developmental paediatrics.

Sophie needed help with her communication, we now understood. With the support of an amazing speech pathologist and supportive educators, a plan was made to meet her where she was at and build her capacity from there. Assessment revealed that she was behind in her expressive (talking) and receptive (listening) language skills, but these alone did not account for all of her difficulties. It was also revealed that she was behind in her pragmatic language abilities too.

Pragmatic language development is all about how we communicate socially, and is a completely separate aspect of language compared to speech and comprehension.[9] It's easy to notice if a child is using as many words as they should for their age, but it's much more challenging to pick up if they understand how to use those words effectively in social settings. Often children who lack these skills can be seen as misbehaving or angry, drawing attention to themselves through behavioural problems. But under the surface, they are essentially being asked to dance without knowing the moves, an experience that would make most of us withdraw or become frustrated. Examples of pragmatic language skills are understanding greetings (hello/goodbye), taking turns in conversation and changing the conversation based on the setting (playground/classroom) or person they are speaking to (child/adult).

Sophie also struggled to understand non-verbal cues, such as facial expressions, which is a common challenge for children who lack pragmatic language skills. This lack of ability to gain non-verbal information along with her pragmatic difficulties meant that without targeted support, Sophie was likely to stall in developing friendships and be well behind her peers by the time she was ready to start school.

Now that we had identified Sophie's various skill gaps, it was time to equip Sophie's parents with the tools to help her. Language enrichment is a really important part of the early environment of children. We have known for decades that children who hear more words, especially words that ask questions or affirm their behaviour, will have a larger vocabulary and greater language skills as they get older.[10] One difficulty in helping children develop their language is that they don't enjoy activities they aren't good at. Lucy and Sam talked about how they'd try every night to read to Sophie, but it only led to outbursts and refusal. This is common in children with language problems, and tends to occur for the same reason that we see in other areas of development – we are setting the bar too high. If my first attempt at weightlifting required me to lift 200 kilograms, I'd never try it again. That's what was happening for Sophie.

Understanding that meant that Lucy and Sam could simplify the books they were reading, starting with picture books with fewer words, and making sure it was fun. They also used picture cards to help Sophie express herself. An apple for food, a glass of water for a drink and a variety of facial expressions for feelings. There is no evidence that supplementing communication with pictures reduces how much children talk, and it is likely to help grow the areas in their brain that process language.[11] People incorrectly think we need to force children to use words or they will become dependent on non-verbal forms of communication such as pointing and other gestures. In truth, we want children to succeed at communicating their needs, so we can start here and then gently extend all of the ways they do this as a secondary step.

The pictures of facial expressions were particularly helpful for Sophie, as their use focused on one of her particular difficulties. Through those pictures, books and modelling by Lucy and Sam, Sophie began to understand when faces were happy, sad and angry. With time, they noticed that Sophie now looked others in the eyes more frequently and for longer, leading to much more shared enjoyment in play, first with adults and then with her peers.

In terms of helping to develop Sophie's expressive language, we asked Lucy and Sam to follow Sophie's lead in communication, reinforcing any form of language by engaging fully with her, asking lots of questions, expanding on what she was saying and exaggerating their expressions to help her learn the rhythm of language. It was wonderful to see an explosion of new words and phrases each time she came to see me in the clinic.

In my most recent appointment with Sophie, Lucy and Sam, we had the chance to assess where Sophie was up to in her social skills and make sure we were all on track. Sophie was back in childcare after first ensuring she was doing well in smaller and more manageable social settings. She was now succeeding at childcare too and learning important social skills such as recognising the emotions of others, sharing and asking for help.

In this appointment, Sam brought up a discussion that we'd had at an earlier session about empathy. He asked how they could support Sophie to build her empathy, now that things were on track with her other social skills. This question gave us a chance to talk about this practically.

Parents have a big influence on how children develop empathy, through multiple pathways. Ensuring we model empathy to our children, partners and others we interact with is a key aspect for children, as they learn to be compassionate by seeing others do it first. Inclusion is an important element of this. A much deeper level of empathy is gained when we can extend it towards all, not just those in our close circle. We can help our children develop this kind of empathy by pointing out similarities we share with others, especially those who may on the surface seem quite different to us, and by helping to foster opportunities for connection, prosocial interactions and diversity in relationships. We should also talk to children about how others may feel about our interactions with them, the good and the bad, such as how to show kindness towards others and offer help when we see someone in need, just as we would want to be helped.

In my consulting room there is a little child-sized table with an assortment of toys, paper and colouring pencils. Despite my adult frame being too big for the chairs, I often feel more comfortable sitting here when younger kids come to see me. One of the easiest things we can do to connect with younger kids is to get down to their level. It is easy to forget how much harder it is to interact with someone when they are towering above you. When Sophie comes to see me now, I spend most of my time at this table connecting with her while I talk with her parents.

All of her parents' efforts shine through in this space too. We pick out the toys together or decide what to draw. She looks at my face to see if I agree and uses the feedback I give her through both my words and my body language to help decide what the toys will do or which colour she will choose to draw with. It is beautiful to see her growth in her social development and hear about her success testing it out in the real world.

Lucy and Sam delight in it too. The last time I saw Sophie, she gave us all a good laugh. We were playing with the toys and I tested her. 'Sophie, could I please use the green truck? It's my favourite.' She quickly dropped the pencils and grabbed the broken truck out of the toy box and began playing with it herself. I asked again, and this time the reply back was a push of the pencil tin in my direction, suggesting I should be satisfied with that option instead, as now she was playing with the truck. Her parents and I shared a chuckle, all well aware that she was just being a typical gorgeous and egocentric toddler.

Key lessons from Chapter 3:

- Social skills are learnt in partnership with others. As parents we guide children in this dance through purposeful and playful interactions. The way they learn to interact with us will echo through their lives in how they treat others and what they expect from them. It is really important that kids enjoy this dance.
- Prosocial skills are the basic steps of positive interactions with others and include empathy, respect, kindness and gratitude. While we often talk about these skills it is much more important that we model these behaviours to them directly, and to others when they are with us.
- Signs that a child might need extra support with their social skills are isolation, a lack of deep friendships, bullying, frequent conflict or no friends their age. Identify the specific social skill they are lacking and help them to develop it until they have overcome that social challenge.

Strategies for parents:

- Observe your children in their social interactions. Ask them about their friendships and talk with their educators about these aspects of their daily lives too.
- Children and teenagers should be succeeding most of the time in their interactions with others, and over time they should be developing deeper and more meaningful relationships within their peer group. If they are frequently having negative social interactions, such as bullying, peer pressure or conflict, or alternatively do not have close connections, it is important to figure out which specific aspect of their social development is struggling.
- Once this specific challenge is found, then they need to be supported at skilling up to overcome it. Things like empathy, understanding facial expressions, conflict resolution and language can all be taught to children through discussion, role modelling, opportunity and feedback. Like everything in this book, it is essential that we do this gently and in partnership with the child.

4. Supporting emotional development is one of our most important roles in guiding children.

Chapter 4

Emotional development

Yvette has always been well ahead in her language development. Her first word was 'Daddy' and her second was 'shoes'. 'Mummy' came just before 'Melfi' (our border collie dog), thankfully. While we have tried hard to enrich her environment as much as we can, so much of her time has been with others. From four months of age, Yvette spent each day in childcare, often one of the first kids dropped off and the last picked up, because Annaliese and I worked long hours with no family around to help. The amazing educators at her childcare deserve a great amount of praise for her development, including her language and social skills.

Childcare can get a bad rap, with some believing incorrectly that research shows it leads to negative outcomes for children. I push back on this in my work for two reasons. First, evidence shows that childcare is often a rich opportunity for children to flourish, especially in their language and social development.[1] Second, many of us have no other choice. I remember a close friend being surprised that we had Yvette in childcare so early and for so long. 'When I have kids I don't want someone else to raise them,' he said. I used my social skills to navigate that conversation carefully. I didn't take it personally – I knew he didn't know how much research has been done about the impact of childcare on child development, and that there are lots of positive outcomes for kids who attend it regularly.

Despite Yvette coming along in leaps and bounds in her language skills (she even corrected me recently when I said a cliff was tall: 'No, Daddy, it's steep'), she still has a vulnerability, one that many kids share. Kids who are bright, especially those who are ahead of their peers in certain areas, are at huge risk of developmental and mental health difficulties because adults often expect too much of them emotionally. I constantly meet teenagers who, because they are articulate and seem mature in many ways, are treated as adults and end up becoming overwhelmed by the expectations placed on them. Just because they are more advanced than other kids their age in their language skills doesn't mean they are also ahead in other aspects of their development, such as emotional regulation. Sometimes, in fact, *because* of their advanced ability in one aspect of their development, they are behind in others. It is common for a child to lean into the success and praise of one skill by focusing on that and miss opportunities to develop in areas they are not as strong in.

Riley was a perfect example of this. Five years old when I met him, he had been forced to grow up too fast. He was brought to me with his grandfather with the support of child protection. We meet many children in the clinic who have child protection involved due to abuse or neglect from their caregivers. This is all too common around the world, with an increased need for these services. My opinion is that children and their families are becoming disconnected from all of the protective aspects of the community they live within, such as extended family, extracurricular activities and cultural traditions. This social isolation in turn leads to worsening mental health in parents, and the result is a devastating impact on children.

Riley hadn't seen his father for years, and his mother struggled with substance abuse and schizophrenia. He had been removed from her care three months earlier and placed with his grandfather, Gus. Gus lived in a caravan in a rough suburb about an hour out of Melbourne, living alone since Riley's grandmother died ten years ago and struggling to make ends meet on a pension. He was delighted to have Riley with him, but he was really worried about him. Riley was in his first year of school, but he had been asked to attend only for limited hours due to emotional difficulties. He had been getting very upset and lashing out at others, to the extent that the school had decided he could only attend for the first two hours each day, leaving at recess. Gus didn't work and was home in the caravan, so he could look after him, but Gus said Riley was getting upset a lot with him too. When I asked what would trigger Riley to become upset, Gus said most of the time he couldn't tell, but being told no was a common one, or any change to plans. The school said the same. Riley was so sensitive to what happened around him that he was breaking down multiple times per day, and Gus, his teachers and the child protection team were all at a loss as to what to do.

Thomas Boyce, a fellow developmental paediatrician, has a beautiful way of describing sensitive children.[2] He talks about how many children are dandelions: they grow with some sun and water, but can do well in most places and are able to handle most weather without a problem. He describes other children as orchids. Changes in water and sun can have a big impact on their growth. Sensitive children like Riley are orchids, and changes and adversity can harm their development and mental health. I love meeting orchids in clinic, and not just because I'm an orchid myself. With the right nurturing, orchids can flourish, perhaps more than dandelions – even those who haven't had the sun and water they needed earlier on in their growth.

How to know if you have a sensitive kid

As we discussed in Chapter 1, sensitive kids are those who have big emotions. The sensitivity is about their responses to what happens around them, and we know new environments, people and experiences can be really challenging for them. Their reactions can seem to come from nowhere or be bigger than expected for what happened; for example, an emotional meltdown over small changes, or shutting down when there is an opportunity to try something new.

I was a sensitive kid and still am a sensitive adult. I will always be an orchid. It took until my thirties to understand how to harness this and care for this aspect of myself. Yvette is an orchid too. Along with

> her red hair, this aspect of my genetics has been passed down to her. I hope to guide her in harnessing and caring for this aspect of identity so that she faces less emotional turmoil than I did growing up and in my early adult life.

Emotional difficulties are by far the number one reason I meet children in the clinic. Amelia and Max, for example, needed help with their emotions. Most of the evidence for supporting younger children tells us that the best way to help them is to build the capacity of the adults around them.[3] For Amelia, we taught her parents how to soothe her, and for Max, we taught his mum how to spot earlier signals that he is dysregulated and how to then guide him towards healthier behaviours. For children Riley's age (five years) and older, however, we can help them build their emotional abilities directly.

With every child I meet in the clinic, after building rapport, my first job is to hear their story. I usually hear about their difficulties first, and then together we search for their strengths. Often these difficulties are tied to the hardest parts of their story. After more than two decades of hearing heartbreaking stories from children and families, it takes a bit to shake me, but Riley's story really tested my ability to remain professional with this vulnerable child.

When I asked about Riley's interests, he told me he loved footy and animals. He and his grandfather were both wearing jerseys for the team they followed, and Riley proudly told me the name of his favourite player. Gus couldn't afford to take Riley to see the games, but each weekend they watched their team on the TV in his caravan. When I asked more about animals, Riley became quiet. Gus said that Riley adored animals, but he was having a hard time thinking about them at the moment. I found out that at his mum's house Riley had lots of pets, including a dog, birds and fish, which he looked after. He was very good at it. When Riley left that home, he was desperate to bring them with him, but they wouldn't fit in with him and Gus. He wanted to visit them each weekend, but his mum cancelled the supervised visits each time at the last minute. Finally Gus took him there, and devastatingly, they found all of the pets had died from a lack of food and water.

I'll never forget the look on Riley's face as I heard that last part. His expression wasn't one of anger or sadness, but acceptance. Riley had experienced so much suffering in his five years that he thought this kind of loss was normal. I wanted to pick him up, look into his eyes and tell him I was sorry in an attempt to bring out the emotions he was feeling about this tragedy, but of course that's not my job in that situation. Gus was already providing emotional support, but what I did do was apologise to Riley about what had happened to his pets and tell him I understood why he was sad and finding it hard to think about animals right now. This story had given an insight into where Riley's difficulty lay – in expressing his emotions.

Emotional development is a broad and complex topic that is hugely misunderstood. As parents and professionals working with children, we need to proactively support our kids' emotional development to guard them against future difficulties.

One of the key things to ensure we teach them is how to seek help when they are drowning in difficult emotions.

Teaching children any skill requires that we ask ourselves two key questions: What specifically are we working on together, and how much support do I need to provide for this child to succeed at it? Take learning to ride a bike, for example. We keep an eye out for signs that a child is ready and then we talk about it excitedly with them. We get a bike small enough for them, maybe a tricycle or one with training wheels, and we prop them up on it, holding them for support. We use encouraging language, and we watch closely for any sign that they are going to fall. If we see it quickly enough, we catch them, if not we help them get up, and gently and lovingly guide them back onto the bike. If the fall was a bad one, we call it a day and tell them how proud we are of them. Helping our kids with their emotional development is exactly the same.

Riley was struggling with his emotional expression. Children who haven't had early support in their emotional development can often be emotionally reactive. They only have one possible response, an outburst of emotions, meaning they go from zero to one hundred in the blink of an eye. For babies like Amelia, this is normal and expected. They haven't had any opportunity to develop the skills and ability to express their emotions. Even though Riley was five years old, he had also missed out on the opportunities to develop his emotions. His mother's substance use and mental illness meant that she likely wasn't able to support him and mostly modelled her own emotional outbursts. Riley hadn't attended any daycare, and his mum kept him home most of preschool. He arrived at primary school completely unequipped to navigate this environment emotionally.

So where did we start? First, I considered his school. I didn't have a problem with Riley being on reduced hours there. Children with behavioural difficulties place such a strain on educators and other children, and they often can't handle a full day at school until they get some help. I see lots of children in this situation. My only request is that these reduced hours have a purpose and an end date for review. The reduction in hours needs to be for a short period of time, to allow the child to succeed during the hours they are at school, build their confidence and therefore their capacity to attend full time.

It turned out Riley was a really social and bright kid. His love of animals demonstrated how caring he could be, and he had picked up his grandfather's sense of humour, cheekily stirring me up in the clinic about how he could beat me at video games with his eyes closed. He was desperate for social connection, and his only friend was a fourteen-year-old boy who lived nearby and had been kicked out of school. They played together each afternoon, not caring about the age difference, as both of them had been removed from a place where they could build friendships with kids their own age. He had also shown his intelligence when he first started at school. He missed so much early education, as his mum didn't take him. Despite limited opportunities to develop his cognitive skills, he was above the expected level on his reading, writing and spelling. Given his social and intellectual strengths, school had the potential to be a place that elevated Riley and further strengthened his self-esteem. Before we could get Riley back to full-time school, however, we needed to work on him succeeding in the hours he was there.

A big step happens in emotional development when kids can put their feelings into words. Having a way to describe how we are feeling provides an opportunity to then build pathways to handle those feelings, especially when they overwhelm us. Our role as adults supporting a child to learn this is to see all emotions as an opportunity for connection and then skill development. Just like when we help them ride a bike, we need to provide the level of support they need to succeed. When a child falls off the bike we know it's not their fault; the hill might be too steep or we backed off with our support too quickly. We should try to respond in the same way when a child struggles emotionally. Seeing emotions as opportunities for connection helps us avoid dismissing them or becoming frustrated. If we fall into that trap, this can lead to kids burying their emotions, just like Riley was doing, until they can't hide them any longer and they erupt – in Riley's case, becoming upset and lashing out at others.

Remember that the main way that our children learn from us is by watching us. The challenge is that how we behave will trump any conversations we have. We may tell them how it is okay to be scared, but if we then belittle others who are scared or hide our own fears, we risk them learning that these emotions are actually not okay. The same goes for how we treat others and ourselves. Conversations about the importance of kindness or self-respect will mean little if we are cruel to others or let people take advantage of us.

Connecting with a child in the hope of understanding and validating their emotions helps to build their ability to accept support and, hopefully, to ask for it in future when they are struggling. It also allows us to help to build their language around emotions, to understand their feelings and the feelings of others, which is a really important skill for future relationships.

When trying to connect with a child it is important we do it with genuine curiosity. You might say, 'I can see you're upset' to show kids that we recognise they are having big feelings and we want to understand. It's hard to demonstrate that same curiosity if you simply tell kids to 'calm down'. Just like with little Max, saying 'I'm here' instead of 'It's okay' doesn't try to hurry them along, and it doesn't dismiss their very real emotions, which might not feel okay. The goal in this moment is to create the space for the child to talk. Any time they do, we should encourage it as it gives us insight into the feelings and thoughts that go along with them. Responding to their own words by labelling the emotions you identify can help to develop their language too. For example, if they say, 'I hate Billy', you might respond with, 'I can see you're angry at Billy' and then explore that feeling with them. That teaches them that when they feel like they do, that's anger.

When responding to a child's emotions, it is important to always validate them, especially the negative ones. We can't help children learn how to navigate emotions like jealousy, anger or sadness if we don't first acknowledge that they exist, or if the child doesn't feel like they can talk to us about those feelings because we don't want to hear it. Many children will need lots of guidance around these difficult emotions, especially those orchid kids who tend to have big emotional reactions to their experiences. These emotions often overwhelm their entire bodies, not just their thoughts, and the heat and tension they experience can be really scary. Sharing our own experiences with difficult emotions can be helpful too, when done in small doses and with open questioning. For example, you might say, 'I know when I don't get the award at work I get annoyed and my heart starts racing. Does anything like that happen for you?' This kind of honesty from us helps kids to learn that they are not alone in struggling with these difficult feelings.

It's a little early to be doing this with Yvette, given her young age, but when you consider how much time I spend talking about emotional development in my work, it's probably no surprise that I sneak discussion of emotions into our play fairly frequently. Antonio, her teddybear that was also mine as a kid, frequently rides the rollercoaster of emotions when we play with him. He gets upset when he isn't picked for the tea party and is sad when Rosie the doll doesn't want to dance with him. He is really happy when the song we sing is about him and jumps for joy when he makes the cut to sleep in Yvette's bed that night. I also broadcast my own emotions, modelling the language to describe them. Our neighbours are probably curious why I'm discussing out loud my frustration when I have a flat bike tyre. Even if we are good at talking directly to children about their emotions, we might forget that they are constantly watching how we deal with our own. If we always pretend everything's okay in front of them, children might grow up thinking something is wrong with them when they can't handle their own feelings, so I choose moments to express my feelings that are age-appropriate for Yvette to understand.

The final step in responding to emotional difficulties is the most challenging: don't fix it. If I come home from a tough day in the clinic and tell Annaliese about it, she knows I only want her to listen. She's got very good at this. (Having an orchid in your life does that to you!) If her response after I told her about a tough day was to immediately tell me that tomorrow will be better or ask if I realise how lucky I am to have the life I do, I'd find it pretty frustrating. Our kids are no different. Listening to them, validating their emotions and helping them to express them is crucial before we get anywhere near helping them deal with those feelings.

When that time does come to help our kids figure out how to improve things, it's important that we guide them towards the solution, but don't try to do it all for them. We often expect older kids to come up with a solution with no support at all, and this too is a mistake. While some teenagers are great at problem solving, many need guidance to go through each of these steps to find an answer. This helps build resilience, too.

With all kids, but especially teenagers, connection is the key. First, we should try to connect with kids, then understand what is going on for them. All emotions are an opportunity to connect, but negative or difficult emotions are signs that we really need to. This won't always be possible, especially with teenagers who withdraw from us, but it's really important we try. We need to show them that we are there, even when it doesn't lead to connection. In terms of understanding, we must try not to come across as judging them or demanding an explanation. Asking questions in an open way and signalling the desire to help can be a useful approach. 'I can see how upset you are. I wonder what you are feeling and why this has made you feel this way. I'm here to help in any way that I can.'

When we get to the problem-solving part, our best chance for it to be effective is if we guide them towards it instead of putting words in their mouth. Saying things like 'What might help you to feel better?' or 'I wonder what could repair what has happened' helps to gently open up these thoughts in their mind. We can then help the make adjustments to the strategy and play a support role in implementing it. In doing so, we show the kids in our lives that we are unconditionally on their side.

In my time with Riley, those of us supporting him, including me, Gus, the child protection team and his educators, found a shared understanding of how best to respond to his emotional difficulties. His previous trauma, his emotional sensitivity and how bright he was helped us understand his specific needs. Given how delayed he was in the area of emotional development, the first thing we worked on was teaching him to seek help. Just like a child who hasn't ridden a bike before, Riley wasn't able to handle his emotions on his own. But from the adults in his life constantly seeing his emotions as opportunities to connect with him and responding with warmth and curiosity, Riley learnt that there was always someone around who he could turn to for help. After months of this he started to express his emotions unprompted, and to explore helpful ways of dealing with them. The school was amazing at using this opportunity to build the emotional development of the whole class, which helped Riley to feel like he wasn't being singled out. They spent weeks learning about feelings and what happens in our bodies when we feel happy, angry or afraid. Riley had a leadership role in this too, frequently demonstrating his language and social skills by talking in front of the class about what happens to our heart, lungs and muscles when we have strong emotions. With time he was back full time at school, succeeding there and he also started playing with a local footy team, to the delight of his grandfather.

If I'm totally honest, I did do one thing outside of my professional role with Riley. The story about his pets kept coming into my mind, and I really struggled to shake it. Animals were something I had connected with Riley about, as I had grown up surrounded by them and learnt about caring for others through this experience. I'd previously worked with a children's farm that was close to where Riley and his grandfather lived, and I knew how much they cared about the kids in their community. One quick phone call was all it took to get him a free membership and an opportunity to meet the team. There, he was able to see others who cared for animals, people who shared that with each other and the broader community, providing a pathway for him to build this strength in himself too. I hope I helped in other ways, but I think that one phone call might have been the best thing I did for Riley. In all of the challenges he was experiencing, he showed me a way to harness his strengths.

Key lessons from Chapter 4:

- Emotions are a big and important part of life, and we learn how to handle them during childhood. It is important that children learn all emotions are okay, especially negative ones, otherwise they are at risk of hiding them or not getting the support they need to learn how to deal with them.
- Our role is to support children to understand their difficult emotions. We should see these emotions as opportunities to connect with our kids, and be curious and validating with a genuine desire to help them without judgement or dismissal. We then help kids figure out ways to express their emotions in a way that does not hurt others.
- A common mistake we can make with difficult emotions is trying to fix them. While well intended, this risks us moving past the experience without our children achieving any growth in their emotional development. If a solution is needed, this step comes after understanding and validating and should be guided by the child.

Strategies for parents:

- When it comes to our children's emotional development, we have three important roles. First in how we respond to them, second in how we model our own emotions and third in how we talk about emotions.
- When responding to emotions, make sure that all are seen as valid and important in life. Put some effort into creating opportunities for emotions like joy, pride and love. Support should be the priority with tough emotions like anger, fear and jealousy, because this is how kids can get better at managing them.
- Openly model your own emotions. We should clearly show how we seek out positive emotions and manage and recover from difficult emotions. This helps our kids learn that both are normal, and that none of us are perfect at it but we're trying to get better.
- Discuss and explore the importance and richness of emotions with your children. The 'suck it up' approach at best limits our emotional growth and at worst further impairs kids who are struggling with difficult emotions and mental illness.

5. Your child's self-esteem now has an impact later in life.

Chapter 5

Self-esteem

There are so many reasons that families bring children to meet me in the clinic. Often in a single day I'll talk about aggression, learning difficulties, bullying, emotional challenges, language concerns, social isolation and trauma. But in all of those children, I almost always worry about one particular factor of their development and mental health: their self-esteem.

Many developmental experts think of childhood and adolescence as being made up of a series of tests. Some describe them as a series of increasingly complex skills that are needed to understand and navigate the world, with the goal being independence.[1] Others talk about key aspects of development such as trust, autonomy and identity.[2] Given the right environment and support, children pass each of these tests successfully, developing the required skills and aspects of development. If they don't, however, they may fail to achieve certain developmental abilities or, perhaps worse, develop dysfunctional skills to compensate.

Many children who are struggling have failed to successfully pass these challenging tests. It may be that they find it difficult to regulate their emotions, understand the perspective of others or restrict impulsive behaviours, all of which can lead to difficulties in daily life. Children who have low or fragile self-esteem are often reluctant to try new things, have big emotional responses to any feedback that isn't completely positive and may even aggressively defend their superiority over others.

Passing these tests is important for another reason, though. Children need to succeed in order to build a healthy level of self-esteem. Self-esteem is the value they see in themselves – their sense of self-worth – and it has an enormous influence on lifelong mental health.[3]

Abbey was seven years old when I met her. She was pretty shy at that first appointment, initially only looking at the ground and not responding to any questions. I always get intrigued when this happens. Part of my brain is listening to the story the parent is telling me, trying to establish a shared understanding of their concerns, the journey so far and what the priorities might be for this family. But another part of my brain is listening for a 'hook'.

Hooks are a form of motivation, a way that I can connect with and help encourage the kids I meet in the clinic. We often know the hooks for the parent or the teacher, but not the child. Parent hooks are often things like wanting their child to flourish and to gain a happier household. Teacher hooks might be wanting to understand why the child is struggling and to gain a calmer classroom. The hooks for kids are always different to those of their parents and teachers, and we don't spend enough time figuring out what these are before launching in with our attempts to change their behaviour. We first need to connect with them and find out why they might want things to be different too.

I started by asking Abbey if she knew why she was here to see me. No response. It's not uncommon for a child who has never met me to avoid answering my questions. I recognise how vulnerable they are in that moment, and I don't push for a response straightaway. I checked with her if it was okay that I asked her mum that question. This time a shoulder shrug came back to me. I took that as progress, said thanks and explained that my job, which I was paid to do, was to help and in the end she would decide if I had done my job well or not. I told her that her mum might tell me some things that she thought weren't going great, but only because I might be able to make them better. Then I told her that if we said anything wrong, I wanted Abbey to correct us, because she was the only one who really knew what was going on. Fleeting eye contact and a nod let me know I could keep going, so I asked her mum how I could help.

Her mum, Sally, told me that Abbey was really struggling academically. She was in Grade 1 at school, but she was at least a year behind in her learning, even though she had thrived in kinder and transitioned well into primary school. During the first few months of school, however, her teachers noticed she wasn't picking up the information as well as other students. Slowly she fell behind in her reading and spelling. It wasn't an issue of effort. She wanted to learn and would try to follow all of the instructions given to her. The teachers said she was a joy to teach and was never disruptive or causing trouble, but they had noticed that Abbey was participating less and less in group activities. She went from often being the first to put her hand up to needing lots of encouragement to attempt an answer out loud. This apparent lack of confidence had been impacting her in the playground too, in terms of socialising with other kids. More often than not, Abbey would just sit and watch the other kids play during breaks. Instead of increasing her participation and confidence at school, which is a big goal that we should have for all kids, Abbey was going in the opposite direction. It was clear to me that her self-esteem was the issue here.

When we are helping kids with their self-esteem, we often make the mistake of aiming for high self-esteem. I'm sure we all grew up with kids who thought quite highly of themselves, and many of us probably know adults like this too. While that level of confidence can seem appealing, the risk with high self-esteem is that it can be really fragile. People with fragile self-esteem often really struggle with any kind of criticism or failure, they may be highly reactive and they may avoid challenges completely out of fear of failure. What we should be aiming for in ourselves and the kids we support is *stable* self-esteem. While self-esteem is not set in childhood, it is built during this period and it can be difficult to shift once it's been low for some time. Being proactive about building a strong and stable sense of self – one that can take constructive feedback on board without it destroying their self-esteem – helps children and adolescents navigate the challenges ahead of them.[4]

Many of the kids I meet in the clinic are struggling due to their self-esteem being fragile or low, and if you are caring for a child with similar issues, all is not lost. There is a great deal that we can do as parents and professionals to rebuild and support self-esteem for our children.

Even though Yvette is much younger than Abbey, I am already trying to guide her towards stable and secure self-esteem. While I often say I am proud of her, I also tell her she should be proud of herself when she succeeds at something such as a puzzle or sharing. Too many children see their self-worth being determined by the praise and acceptance of others, leading to a fragility when they are not told how great they are. It also makes them vulnerable to taking on board unfair criticism, such as being told they are less than others due to their appearance or abilities. From a young age we can help our kids to see that their opinion of themselves is more valuable than the opinions of other people.

I also try to separate her efforts from who she is as a person. When a child is misbehaving, it is helpful to separate the behaviour from the child, for example, by saying a specific behaviour is mean instead of saying the child is mean. We need to do the same when they succeed, so that children understand that our care and support is unconditional, and 'good' or 'bad' behaviour will not challenge our love or support of them. This protects them from feeling like they are not good enough or that they need to perform well constantly to keep us on side. Separating the child from their behaviour when they are succeeding is called 'process praise'.[5] Instead of telling Yvette she is so smart or good at drawing, which is called 'person praise', I try to remind myself to reinforce her effort: 'You worked so hard on that drawing and it looks beautiful.'

Another thing I do is make sure that Yvette knows she is valued and needed in our family. She has roles that only she does, such as helping me to shave, feeding the worms and watering the strawberries. While these might seem a bit silly or lighthearted, I'm trying to show her how important she is to the family. This is a sense that every child needs, not just for the security of their self-esteem but also for any future challenges to their mental health. When we are really struggling, a sense of being valued and needed by others can carry us through.

The final pillar of how I try to build Yvette's self-esteem is with what I call 'sanctuaries'. All kids need them, and every day in the clinic I help build them with families. Sanctuaries are like rituals – activities we do or places that we go together that are only for joy. They have to happen frequently, consistently and be untouchable. Families need to have sanctuaries for all members, and each child needs to have them for just themselves and each parent.

Each person needs to genuinely enjoy the sanctuary to really harness the joy within the time together. Taco Tuesdays are no good if someone doesn't like Mexican food, and playing video games with Mum won't become a sacred family ritual if she doesn't enjoy them too. The most important aspect of the chosen sanctuaries is that they are untouchable. No matter what else is going on in our lives, the sanctuary remains. It is in these really difficult moments that we can prove our unconditional love for our kids. These activities are, sadly, often the first to slip away in busy households, but they are way more important than homework and eating our vegetables. Knowing that you are enjoyed and celebrated by your family is a cornerstone of healthy development and mental health.

I still remember one of my sanctuaries with my mum, who died when I was in my early twenties. I didn't see her much growing up because she worked three jobs, but somehow she made it to some of my extracurricular activities consistently. In primary school I was chosen to be in the boys choir. My mum would take me to rehearsals and afterwards we would walk through the park nearby to the fairy tree. This old tree has carved and painted fairies up its trunk, and we would sit there as she told me their stories, carrying on the narrative from the previous week's visit. Decades later, that sanctuary is a special memory of my mum. On the day we took Yvette and then Charlie home from the hospital after being born, we visited that tree to introduce them to my mum, that sanctuary echoing from my childhood into theirs. I think these echoing memories are what many of us are aiming for with our kids, and these stories of love and connection stay with them long after we've gone.

So could I teach Abbey and her family these three methods – praising behaviour, looking at roles in the family, and identifying or creating sanctuaries – to help Abbey with her self-esteem? Abbey was the middle child, with a nine-year-old brother, Marcus, and a four-year-old sister, Charlotte. Marcus was really bright and doing well at school; he was just like his dad, Thomas, who was an engineer. The two of them were really close and loved building things together in the shed. Charlotte was a ball of energy. She always seemed happy and outgoing, talking, playing and having fun. I could see how much everyone in the family loved Charlotte, but also that she often received all of the attention from her parents, regardless of what else was going on.

With Abbey listening, Sally and I talked about how Abbey wasn't getting the same amount of attention as Marcus and Charlotte were from Sally and Thomas. Thomas had a real connection with Marcus, and Charlotte filled any time and space that there was in their busy home. Sally mentioned how much she adored Abbey, saying she wished that she had more protected time with her. As we spoke I could see Abbey was paying attention and slowly warming up. She agreed with Sally when she said that Charlotte takes up a lot of her time and laughed when her little sister was described as the boss of the family.

Now felt like the right time to ask the two questions I ask every child I meet in the clinic: what do they like and what are they good at? With help from Sally, Abbey told me she really likes drawing and painting, often made-up animals and people. Dragons and fairies were her favourite. Sally showed me some of the drawings she'd taken photos of on her phone. When I asked Abbey what she was good at, though, she gave me the same shrug as before. Her mum jumped in with a long list of things, but I could see Abbey didn't believe them.

Every day I meet children who can't answer one or both of those questions, and this is good information about the state of their mental health. Answers to the second question – what are you good at? – tend to fall away first, as kids who are struggling start to feel overwhelmed by any failure in their life. They start to believe they are not good at anything. And if this is left unaddressed, answers to the first question fall away too. A lack of interest in things, especially things they used to love, is a core symptom of mental illness in children.

I'd been given a hook, though, and I ran with it. I wanted to learn more about Abbey and her creative skills, especially how frequently she got to practise them. Sally said she wasn't sure about during school hours, but she had noticed that Abbey was drawing less often at home. When Abbey was younger, Sally and Thomas had always found the time sit with her, but now it was really tough. The time they did have focusing on her was spent on reading and writing after school, which was a real battle. Often it led to Abbey becoming upset and then refusing to keep trying, a really common story in kids who are falling behind in their learning at school. A big aspect of building skills requires having enough positive self-esteem to attempt something. Abbey had stopped trying in class and the playground due to her declining self-esteem, losing faith in her efforts ever paying off. So many kids give up trying because it ends up making them feel like a failure. While Sally and Thomas were trying to help, the shift of focus from her strengths (her drawing and painting) to her weaknesses (her reading and writing) was weakening her self-worth.

With time, we learnt that Abbey had inattentive sub-type attention deficit hyperactivity disorder (ADHD). She was sitting in class trying her hardest, but wasn't able to take in the information the teacher was providing. Even though she wasn't hyperactive – the classic image of someone with ADHD – under the surface she was struggling to concentrate. This type of ADHD is much more common in girls, and the lack of hyperactivity is the reason we miss diagnosing it so often.[6]

With 5–10 per cent of children meeting clinical criteria for ADHD, there are enough children who do have the hyperactivity part to keep educators busy.[7]

ADHD

ADHD has two core components: hyperactivity and impulsivity, and inattention.[8]

Signs of hyperactivity and impulsivity include feeling restless, difficulty sitting still or waiting their turn, excessive talking and interrupting others. These symptoms usually emerge around four years of age and peak at around eight years of age. Many teenagers won't demonstrate these difficulties.

Signs of inattention include struggling to maintain focus, seeming to not listen, careless mistakes, an inability to complete tasks, losing things frequently, being poorly organised, avoiding difficult tasks and being easily distracted. These difficulties usually emerge later, around nine years of age.

There are three important things to remember:

First, the above symptoms and signs must impact function. I experience many of these difficulties listed, especially the inattention to signs, but they don't significantly impact how I function in my life.

Second, you don't have to have both hyperactive/impulsive and inattentive symptoms to meet diagnostic criteria. Many children with ADHD only have difficulties in one of the two groups of symptoms.

Third, and maybe most importantly, ADHD is not an emotional problem. It is an executive function problem that can cause emotional difficulties (e.g. feeling frustrated because of losing things) or mean that kids struggle to deal with their emotions (react quickly when angry because of being impulsive). We run the risk of dismissing emotional difficulties when we think they are a part of ADHD, but children with ADHD are at an increased risk of emotional difficulties and if they are present, we should always search for a reason why that isn't ADHD.

I love meeting children with ADHD because they are often just like Abbey, really creative. Creativity needs you to be distractible and think differently to others. Artists find and create beauty in the world that no one else has before them, and many of the most famous creators of history are believed to have had ADHD (Leonardo da Vinci and Albert Einstein, for example). The challenge with ADHD is that it is really hard to turn off this sensitivity to distraction, especially when you're being asked to do something you're not very interested in or good at.

The key to helping kids with ADHD is the same as every other aspect of what I do in the clinic: finding the right accommodations and working on skill development.[9] Accommodations are what we can do to make it easier for kids to succeed. We don't ask kids who need glasses to try harder to see, we get them glasses. Similarly, if kids are struggling with other aspects of their daily functioning, we need to find ways to help them.

Accommodations need to be specific to the child too. Just like there are lots of different prescriptions for glasses, support needs to be tailored to the needs of the individual child. Sometimes we make the mistake of thinking there is a one-size-fits-all approach for diagnoses like ADHD. For example, not every child with ADHD needs to sit at the front of the class to be able to concentrate, even though you might think removing as many distractions as possible is the best way forward. Many of them need to be at the back, actually, where the low-level noise coming from all the kids sitting in front of them helps them to remain engaged with the teacher, who is at the front of the classroom.

When it comes to looking at skill development for kids with ADHD, remember that this needs to be tailored too. ADHD is a type of neurodiversity in how the executive function part of our brain works, which has three main aspects.[10] The first is impulse control – this is why many children with ADHD can't help but interrupt in class or casual conversation. They need to be taught how to control that urge gently, with lots of support. The second aspect is mental flexibility – the ability to adapt how we act based on changing information. Kids who struggle with this often find it hard to adapt their behaviour after transitioning from one environment to another. The classic example is a child coming back to the classroom from the playground still radiating energy in their voice, movement and emotions. The third aspect is working memory. This part of executive function helps us to hold a number of pieces of information in our short-term memory to then perform a task.

This concept of working memory was the main reason that Abbey was so far behind and becoming discouraged from trying, contributing to her low self-esteem. She wasn't impulsive or hyperactive, and she tried her hardest to listen to what the teacher said and complete the activities being set. She didn't struggle with her mental flexibility, understanding that she needed to adapt based on the information that came to her from the environment. Where she did struggle though was in understanding multi-step instructions.

Each morning after breakfast, Sally would ask Abbey to get her stuff for school and meet her at the car. Abbey always forgot something, either her lunch, school hat or water bottle. The same thing was happening in class. The teacher would explain the steps needed to carry out the classwork, but then find that Abbey had missed part of it or done one aspect incorrectly. No matter how many times she was told, she struggled with these simple instructions, which the other kids found easy to complete. Unless we helped her develop her skills in this part of her executive functioning, the gap between her and her peers was going to keep widening, further deteriorating her self-esteem.

Like lots of creative kids, Abbey wasn't great at following verbal instructions, preferring to learn visually. She succeeded more with written instructions that she could refer back to, as they helped her to access the working memory part of her brain more easily. Together with the help of a wonderful teacher, Sally and Thomas picked a few things to focus on as a family. At home it was the morning routine, while at school it was individual reading activities. The step-by-step details were decided as a team for both the home and school priorities, and then they built visual instruction plans with the help of Abby's artistic talent.

Two important aspects existed on each of the plans, a check-in and a signal. The check-in began by asking how everyone was feeling, followed by calming activities if needed, to settle any difficult feelings and prepare for the task ahead. The signals were a way for Abbey to indicate that she needed more support. It is helpful for these signals to be non-verbal, as they protect the child from feeling like they are drawing too much attention to themselves, especially in a classroom. For Abbey, the signal at school was for her to put her hand out, palm facing down and moving side to side to show that things were a little wobbly. Her teacher would see this and know Abbey needed a reminder about the instructions or support with the task at hand. At home, she could use a verbal signal, such as saying, 'I'm feeling wobbly.'

The two plans also needed to have specific steps. At home, Abbey's steps were helping to prepare breakfast, picking out school clothes, showering and brushing teeth, getting dressed and then packing her school bag. At school, the steps were confirming that she understood the reading task, checking the book matched the one on the board and finding the right page, holding a stress ball while reading, highlighting three important words on each page and taking a break between each page. Abbey drew a little illustration for each step in the two plans, and kept her home plan in her bedroom and the other on her school desk.

At first Abbey needed help with each step, but quickly her parents and teachers noticed that she needed less and less support to succeed. Frequent monitoring and discussion showed the plans were working as Abbey used the visual cues to reinforce each aspect of the task she was focused on. That alone wasn't going to help with her self-esteem, though.

Everyone involved in helping Abbey worked hard to make sure their language consistently separated behaviours from who Abbey was as a person. When she was daydreaming or forgetful, they could gently point this out and ask what might help, which allowed her to be open to support without feeling criticised. Her family also really prioritised showing her how important she was to the daily functioning of the family. She helped her mum make lunches in the morning and her dad set the table for dinner each night. This gave her an opportunity for her to feel that she was an integral part of the family and also build her working memory skills in this supported environment.

Along with the shift in language and support in strengthening all aspects of her self-esteem, Abbey needed sanctuaries with each of her parents, and eventually her siblings too. Ideally these would be things that would help her feel good about herself. The best scenario is when the child decides what the sanctuary will be, and Abbey proved that right this time too. After I'd explained what sanctuaries were, we all agreed that Abbey and her parents would come back with a few ideas. At that next appointment, Abbey delightedly told me that now she was teaching her dad how to paint. They would set aside an hour each Sunday to get out the paint, brushes and paper, and

Abbey would proudly show him how to create wonderful fairies and dragons. It was a beautiful way to reinforce their relationship and give her opportunities to succeed at something. A big part of self-esteem comes from succeeding at something specific that you see as a part of your identity.[11] Abbey was back being an artist.

With her mum, Abbey found a sanctuary in helping to plan their upcoming summer holiday. This one got bonus points because it also helped her with her working memory in a fun way. Sally would help her decide the bit of the holiday that needed planning, then guide her to come up with the steps for each part of the bigger task. This teamwork was also blurring into other parts of the week, like the food shopping and the chores roster, with great success, further strengthening the important role Abbey played in her family.

I get to catch up with Abbey pretty rarely these days. She's now ahead of where she should be academically, and she's thriving socially at school. While Charlotte is still the boss of the house, Abbey now has protected time with both her parents and knows that she plays an important role in the family. I still love seeing her though, as she brings in artwork that she's recently completed, as well as some of her dad's, giggling as we joke that one day he might be as good as her at painting.

Key lessons from Chapter 5:

- A secure self-esteem protects us against feeling worthless when we face rejection or failure. All children need to be supported in developing a strong sense of worth, because how we feel about ourselves is often built in our interactions with others.
- It is important that we support and praise effort and growth, not success. Otherwise children are vulnerable to feeling that their value is tied to their achievements. This can lead to kids feeling worthless when they fail, or them intentionally avoiding anything where they might fail, such as school or sport.
- A sense of being valued by those around us is essential for secure self-esteem. Families can help create this by building sanctuaries that harness the child's strengths and interests. Having a purpose and experiencing joy with others is an essential aspect of mental health.

Strategies for parents:

- Self-esteem is built during childhood through interactions with others – most importantly us. The goal is to make sure our children know we unconditionally love and support them to protect their self-worth.
- Outlets for expression and growth help to ensure kids feel valued in who they are. Two questions can help with this: what do they enjoy and what do they believe they are good at? Both questions should have multiple answers, and you can help create opportunities for them to experience these activities frequently. This shields them from low self-esteem when working on harder skills to achieve or abilities they do not master immediately.
- When we are working on any skill, it is important that children see it as a partnership in which we support them to get better at something together. Talk about why it will benefit them and those around them, for example, saying that we work towards growth so that children experience more joy and connection in their daily lives at school and home.

6. Anxiety begins in early childhood and should not be ignored.

Chapter 6

Anxiety

In the early 2000s I was working on an adult psychiatric ward in a big public hospital as part of my medical training. It was one of my first experiences caring for patients with severe mental illness, and it was a real turning point in my career.

One of the patients in the ward, Brian, had been admitted in a very agitated state after experiencing a psychotic episode. Brian had a long history of anxiety, trauma and social isolation, and he ended up being on the ward for a long time. In the beginning he had to be sedated daily, but gradually he improved and he ended up being able to have conversations about his feelings in a healthy way. I got to spend quite a bit of time with Brian and loved getting to know him and hearing about his background. By the time he was discharged, he was talking positively about wanting to get his life back on track, reconnect with his family and remain engaged with therapy.

After Brian left, I commented to a nurse that it was great to see him doing so well and that I hoped the treatment lasted and he wouldn't need to come back ever again. The nurse looked at me with a tired expression and said, 'He'll definitely be back. Like most of these patients, it's not a question of if he'll come back, but how soon.'

The nurse wasn't trying to be unkind, they were simply being a realist. As I soon came to realise, adult mental illness is so debilitating and under-resourced that many professionals working with patients feel hopeless about the situation. Child mental health has similar problems but with one major difference: there is so much hope.

What, I wondered, would have been the outcome if someone had intervened when Brian was a kid? Would they have been able to help him avoid the awful experiences he went through as an adult? It was at that point that I decided I was going to focus on the root of the issue to help all those young Brians out there and change the course of their lives. This book is an extension of that commitment.

Over 50 per cent of adult mental illness begins in childhood, and the sooner it is identified and treated, the greater chance we have of making sure those children don't experience ongoing problems.[1] The problem is, however, that we miss so many early signs that a child is struggling. Think about how hard it is for us as adults to understand and share our own challenging emotions. For children it is much harder, as their brains are still developing intellectually, emotionally and socially.

One of the key things they struggle with is anxiety. In fact, more children and adults suffer from anxiety than any other mental illness, including depression.[2] On that adult psychiatric ward where I met Brian all those years ago, I was taught by a leading psychiatrist named Dr Basil Bunting, who described the experience of having anxiety in the most vivid way I've heard. He told us to imagine we were walking through a jungle. 'Your heartbeat is slow,' he said, 'your breathing is shallow and your muscles are relaxed as you enjoy the beautiful surrounds and relaxing birdsong. Then, all of a sudden, you see a tiger. Your nervous system kicks into gear, triggering your flight or fight response even before you are really aware that the tiger is there. Nerves and stress hormones fire through your entire body, making your heart race, breathing rapid and deep and your muscles tense ready for action. All of this happens before you have the emotional experience of fear, as your brain stem circuitry takes milliseconds to get ready for action. The experience (tiger) leads to the emotion (fear), which drives the behaviour (to run). This automatic alarm system is the reason our ancestors survived. They had to be on high alert for tigers, otherwise they became lunch!' We all chuckled as he perfectly balanced story-telling and science.

Unfortunately this same system that keeps us alive when faced with life-or-death situations is the system that causes the leading mental illness in adults and children all over the world: anxiety. Clinical anxiety, at its core, is the experience of tigers that aren't really there. So many kids experience debilitating anxiety every day and for them, the tigers are real. Telling kids there is no tiger not only doesn't help, it often increases their anxiety that they are alone in facing their fears.

Common signs of anxiety in children

Anxiety is a normal emotional response to many situations and can be an appropriate and helpful part of life. It becomes concerning when it has a negative impact on how well a person functions or their quality of life. Anxiety occurs in approximately 7 per cent of children and teenagers.[3]

Symptoms of anxiety include:

- withdrawal and avoidance
- anger and outbursts
- trouble falling asleep or frequent waking through the night
- always needing reassurance
- trouble concentrating
- changes in appetite
- physical symptoms such as headaches, nausea, tummy pain, dizziness and muscle cramps.

There are also many other forms of anxiety. These have additional signs, and include separation anxiety, social anxiety, selective mutism, specific phobia, panic disorder and obsessive compulsive disorder.

Signs that anxiety has reached a concerning level are restlessness, fatigue, difficulty concentrating, irritability, sleep difficulties and muscle tension.

Very few kids can say they are anxious and many will either withdraw, become irritable or complain of feelings in their body such as headaches or tummy pain.

Phillip was a ten-year-old boy who had been sent to see me due to difficulty leaving his house. He lived with his mum, Joanna, father, Chris, and older brother, Jesse, who was sixteen. Like Abbey, Phillip wasn't able to talk to me at that first appointment. In fact, his mum told me he rarely spoke to anyone, and it had been a huge effort just to get him into the clinic that morning to see me. She said that Phillip had been a really happy and active child with no significant concerns up until about two years ago. Looking back, she and her husband noticed that the first signs were occasional tummy aches before school. Initially they thought something might be wrong with his digestive system, so they took Phillip to see their GP. All the tests came back normal, but the tummy aches got worse. Then they tried ignoring them, hoping with time he would stop mentioning them, gently reassuring him when he persisted that the doctor had said nothing was wrong. Within a couple of months Phillip wasn't able to get out of bed in the morning, missing the first part of every school day. Then he started missing entire days and then weeks at a time due to tummy aches and tiredness.

When I first met Phillip, he had missed an entire year of school. Not only that, he could no longer leave the house, often only eating meals in his room, playing video games and watching cartoons. His parents were at a loss as to how they could turn things around. They missed their happy and chatty boy who loved school and his friends there.

We often think of anxiety as a problem teenagers have, but in fact it commonly begins much earlier, as it did in Phillip. All children need to experience fear and worries to learn to handle and resolve these types of experiences, but if children don't manage to navigate these fears successfully, it can impact their mental health.

During the first few years of life, separation from caregivers and interactions with strangers often trigger fear in children. In toddlers this is usually not concerning, but when observed in school-age children it can mean support is required. Selective mutism, a form of anxiety in which children will not speak in certain environments, is usually seen in children before they start school, and needs to be approached from a mental health, not a speech, perspective.[4]

In school, the need to fit in can lead to performance anxiety and worries of peer rejection.

Separation anxiety, where children struggle to separate from their primary caregivers, is another form of clinical anxiety affecting children who are on average seven years old.[5] It also needs to be approached carefully to avoid mental difficulties later in life. Even the teenagers we meet in the clinic who have generalised anxiety, social anxiety or panic attacks, often first started to struggle during primary school.

Helping children learn to understand these feelings and come up with healthy ways to deal with them requires specific skill development. We need to help them identify feelings of fear and worry, teach them words to describe these feelings and communicate them to others, and then learn ways to process these experiences that allow the child to succeed in their daily activities and relationships.

Cognitive behavioural therapy (CBT)

CBT is one of the main approaches we use to treat mental illness. While it isn't always the best or only option, it is evidence-based and useful for you to understand so that you can explore what works for your child.[6] I'll quickly outline it here as it's so useful in treating anxiety.

The first step in CBT is called 'psychoeducation'. That might sound a little daunting, but it simply means giving the child and their carers a better understanding of what is happening to them from a scientific point of view. The description Dr Basil Bunting gave of the tiger in the jungle and our physiological response to anxiety is an exercise in psychoeducation.

The second aspect is symptom control. While this is different for everyone, the general principles are helpful to understand. As we've discussed, anxiety is a triggering of nerves and hormones in our bodies that activates the fight or flight response. What we need to find out when a child has anxiety is what feelings they get when that system gets triggered and what helps to switch it off. Strategies such as deep breathing or muscle contractions and relaxations are really helpful ways to take control of the sensations that tell us we are anxious. With support, kids can become aware of these feelings from a very early age and learn to respond.

The third component of CBT is cognitive restructuring, which is developing new ways of thinking about the things that trigger anxiety in our kids.

The fourth aspect is exposure, where we gently guide children back into situations and environments that previously caused anxiety.

The fifth and final aspect is relapse prevention. One of the biggest risk factors of mental illness is a previous episode, which is why all children and adults who have experienced challenges with their mental health should be supported to proactively work to avoid future episodes, rather than simply breathing a sigh of relief that it has resolved.

Looking into the cause of anxiety is like searching for a tiger. While we can't see the tiger, the child can show us exactly where it is. Once we understand the bodily sensations that children who are anxious experience, we can then use them as signs that the tiger is around. For Phillip, it was clear that the tiger was at school. For many children, the reason that tigers pop up in these environments is due to being overwhelmed by the social and performance aspect of school. From around eight or nine years of age, children start to compare themselves to their peers in an attempt to fit in. School can be a really daunting experience, too, as children start to participate in more obvious forms of evaluation such as presentations and tests. This was when Phillip started to get his symptoms of anxiety. At first it was the night before a school presentation, but then it progressed to any school day due to the fear of being asked to answer a question in class. Phillip had no intellectual or learning concerns, but this didn't fix his fear of failure and social rejection. With time he was so afraid of being overwhelmed and rejected that it had escalated to being unable to leave the house.

There was another reason Phillip struggled to leave home: his dad, Chris. Chris had previously worked in a timber yard in a physically demanding role. You could still see that strength in his physique, but I noticed he had difficulty getting up out of one of the consulting room chairs. He told me he had injured himself a few months before Phillip started to struggle with anxiety, and that he hadn't been able to work for about two and a half years.

For children who are struggling to attend school, there is often an unintentional reinforcer at home. It could be a parent who is struggling with mental illness or, in Phillip's case, a physical disability, or a situation like domestic violence. The injury meant that Chris had gone from working long hours six days a week to always being home. He and Phillip were very close, and we discovered that the opportunity to spend more time with his dad, where Phillip felt lots of comfort and safety, made it even harder for him to move towards situations that caused anxiety, such as school and being out in public.

People are often tempted to make kids with mental illness face what they fear – a strategy known as 'exposure'. I think the expectation is that after a pep talk or a break from the situation, the child will be better able to deal with it. Exposure, however, should not be the first step in managing an anxiety-invoking situation, and telling Phillip he needed to be back in school would have only increased his anxiety.

We didn't need to sever his desire to be with his dad to get him back at school. Instead, we guided him to recognise the signs in his body that signalled his anxiety. This awareness of what our body is telling us is called 'interoception'.[7] For Phillip, this was nausea and a tightness in his tummy. For others it might be the awareness of their heart racing, a headache, feeling hot or a tingling sensation in parts of their body.

Once we'd identified Phillip's early signs of anxiety, the next step was to figure out what helped to *control* those feelings by switching off the fight or flight response. Phillip liked music and found deep breathing calming, so when he started to feel sick or the tight feeling in his stomach, we asked him to find a calm place and go through some breathing exercises that we taught him to help calm his nervous system down. Unlike Max in Chapter 2, Phillip, at age ten, was skilled enough in his development that he could start to use these techniques on his own to give him back his sense of control over those overwhelming experiences. He would take a deep, slow breath in, pause, and then slowly breathe out, focusing on the air moving through his nose and the rise and fall of his tummy. If this strategy didn't resolve his anxiety within five to ten minutes, he would then listen to music somewhere on his own until he felt calm again. We also set up sessions with a psychologist to help address some of his concerns about performance, fitting in and not being with his dad.

After many weeks of practice, it was time for exposure. Even though we had taken some time to work up to this, it is still easy to go too fast with this step. We need to play the long game and gently reintroduce a child to their triggers or triggering environments with lots of support and control. For Phillip, this meant starting with leaving the house and socialising at home, rather than diving straight into a full day at school. We decided together that he would go to see a movie with his dad, then have a friend over to play video games. As he built up his confidence and we decided he was ready to be back at school, he attended in gradually increasing visits, with a low expectation of participation. The class took the opportunity to learn about anxiety, further expanding the psychoeducation component of Phillip's path back to succeeding at school. This also helped with what's called 'relapse prevention', meaning the entire class was better prepared to provide support if anyone showed signs of anxiety.

I should note here that mainstream school is not perfect for all children. While children need opportunities to be guided in their development and no professional does that better than teachers, many children struggle with aspects of schooling that mean they can't succeed in these environments.

Phillip was not one of these children, however, and I was confident that by walking through each step in the path to recovery, we could get him back there successfully. Phillip now attends full time, and he and his teacher have a subtle signal for him to use when he's feeling anxious so that he can leave the class without raising too much attention. He heads to the wellbeing room, where he practises breathing exercises and listens to music, sometimes with the help of his amazing well-being lead Rebecca, other times by himself. He is also seeing his friends, participating in the family and getting to play video games with his dad every weekend.

Key lessons from Chapter 6:

- Feeling anxious is a common and helpful part of life, and all children will experience it to a certain degree. Like all emotions, experiencing anxiety during childhood is an opportunity for kids to be supported in learning how to deal with it.
- Anxiety becomes concerning when it happens frequently and leads to difficulties functioning at home or school. Common triggers can be separating from a caregiver, social interactions and environments where judgement may occur (e.g. the classroom).
- When children are showing excessive anxiety, it is important to support them to understand these feelings and how to manage them. It is different for each child, but management often involves a child learning and practising ways to settle their nervous system, such as deep breathing, tensing and relaxing muscles or listening to music.

Strategies for parents:

- Helping everyone in the family to learn about anxiety is a really great way to build mastery of our feelings, especially the difficult ones. Understanding what can trigger worry and fear and what happens in our body when these feelings happen helps to know when it's present, but also shows kids it's okay.
- When children do become anxious, we must make sure we never dismiss it. Leaving a child to face their fears on their own will worsen those feelings, and risks that they won't tell you about them in the future.
- We should all be constantly learning what works best to help calm us in these tough moments. All children need guidance with this, and it is different for every child. Common approaches tap into calming down the alarm system in our body. Moving to less stimulating spaces helps to settle the alarm in many children, and activities like deep breathing help us to focus on our bodies and the present moment. This can be done from a young age.

7. By prioritising relationships, we can help children learn about respect.

Chapter 7

Respect

I've been asked thousands of questions over the years, but I've made an observation about the one I'm asked most frequently that I find fascinating: it changes slightly depending on who is doing the asking. Mothers ask why their child doesn't *listen* to them. Fathers ask how they can make their child *respect* them. Educators ask how to deal with a child's opposition and refusal to *do as they're told*. In essence, though, they're all asking about how to achieve harmony through authority (the adult) and compliance (the child).

Before we explore this topic, it's important to spend a moment thinking about what we are aiming for as parents and professionals supporting children. One main goal might be to give our kids the best guidance possible to meet the challenges of life. Tough parents might use this as a reason to come down hard on kids: 'Life isn't fair, so they may as well learn that now.' But the problem is that before we can teach anyone anything we need to *connect* with them. A great example of this can be seen in the film *Batman*. When Batman's a child, he's asked by his father, 'Why do we fall, Bruce?' Batman doesn't know the answer so his father provides it for him: 'So we can learn to pick ourselves up.' This approach to developing the skill to overcome adversity lacks one essential component, though: the relationship between parent and child. For all of his crime-fighting skills, Batman saw threats everywhere, could not be his true self and trusted almost no one. He learnt about discipline but lacked the support of others.

The fact is that we learn nothing in isolation. Riding a bike, learning to talk and emotional regulation all need someone to show us how. We fall in childhood not so we can learn to pick ourselves up, but to have someone there to help us up until we can do it on our own.

My goal is that Yvette and Charlie see me as a source of unconditional love and support long after they become adults. I want them to see me as a person who listens to them, tries to understand their experience and faces any challenge by their side. Many parents I meet in the clinic and the community tell me that this is their goal too and their kids know this. When I ask how their children know this, the answer is usually 'because I tell them all the time'. However, the tricky bit is that kids don't know we unconditionally love and support them because we *tell* them, they know it because we *show* them, over and over again. That is much harder. But if we want our children to follow the rules we want them to follow, we need to prioritise the relationship first, to build and maintain trust and respect.

For Yvette, I try to make sure the relationship always comes before the rules. The first step is creating connection at every possible opportunity outside of moments of pressure. It is about being truly delighted by the children in our lives. After keeping our kids safe and secure, I think this is the most important thing we can do for them. Multiple times per day, Yvette and I sing and dance together, play silly games and build rituals purely for the sake of fun. I'm starting to do this with Charlie too. I'm not doing it because I'm some kind of superdad, but because every day when I meet families in crisis, I get a reminder about how important this type of connection is.

The second step is creating connection *during* moments of pressure, which only works if you've succeeded in the first step. A moment of pressure might be a child ignoring you, being defiant or actively challenging your authority. I'm not talking about a child who is completely overwhelmed, where their limited development means that much of the support needs to be provided without words. Here, I'm talking about those moments when we clash with our children over everyday issues, where we want to find a better response than 'because I said so'. Going into battle with our kids can become a habitual way of interacting with them and can be a difficult cycle to break, but we need to listen, try to understand their perspective, gently give them ours and try to find a solution together. When this doesn't work with a child who has age-appropriate skills in thinking and reasoning, it's because the relationship needs work, not the rules.

In the thousands of kids I've met, Omar will always stand out. For a twelve-year-old boy, he had an impressive amount of confidence. He introduced himself and shook my hand, sat down and spread out in a chair, making himself comfortable well before his mum even entered the room. To be fair, his confidence was somewhat justified. He was a good-looking kid with a sharp wit. Unfortunately not everyone saw it that way. His mother, Fatima, smiled at me when I asked how I could help. 'How long do you have?' was her response. Omar laughed, and I was starting to see a nice similarity in mother and son already.

Fatima told me how she loved Omar, just as she loved all five of her children, but he was too much. 'He never listens, always answers back and doesn't help out around the house.' Omar was the oldest child in their family. His father wasn't around much, so there was a lot of work every day for a single parent to try and keep on top of. 'It's not just me either, doctor,' Fatima said. She went on to tell me that Omar was talking back to his teacher and thought he was too smart to be at school anyway. She told me that his grades were okay but he should be doing better. He had friends and played soccer with them once a week. He wasn't getting into any serious trouble, but she was worried that he was too selfish.

I listened, nodded and summarised what Fatima had told me. Then I asked Omar what he thought about the things his mum was saying. Straight away he replied, 'She's wrong. She doesn't know what she's talking about.' I could tell he believed what he was saying. As bright as he was, the only perspective he could see was his own. He was behind in one really important part of his development, but we were going to help him catch up.

In Chapter 3, we discussed how we can guide children to develop empathy. This skill is one in which we try to understand the emotional experience of another person. But what about when it isn't our emotions but our perspective that we want kids to learn? Omar wasn't clashing with his mum and teachers because he didn't have empathy for them, it was because he couldn't see their thinking and reasoning. This understanding of another person's perspective is called theory of mind, and it is an essential skill that benefits cognitive growth and social relationships.[1]

Theory of mind first emerges before one year of age. Infants start to understand that other people are different to them when they hand us objects from around eight months of age. Studies have even shown that they will preference handing over toys that are new to the other person, even if that toy isn't new to the infant.[2] This shows us that they are starting to think about other people having a different experience to their own, but it's very early days.

Then, a few months after their first birthday, they start showing us things purely for us to experience them too. This is called protodeclarative pointing, and it signals that their development of theory of mind is on the right track.[3] An example of this might be pointing at a puppy so we see it and enjoy it too, as opposed to directing us to something they want us to get for them. They want us to join in, not because it benefits them but to share the moment, and this experience builds connections and brain growth in the social centre of our brain.

Between the ages of three and five, there is a big burst of growth in this area, and so much of the research into theory of mind has focused on this period.[4] The exciting part is that there is so much we can do during these early years to help children acquire this skill sooner than typical and at a higher level.

False belief

In the 1980s, researchers developed a test to see if children had acquired the ability to understand how the experience and, more importantly, the thinking of others are different to their own. It's called the false-belief task.[5] Many versions of it exist now, but let's use a common childhood experience as an example. As a child, you see a tin of chocolates and get excited. You open the tin to sadly discover that instead of being full of chocolates, it contains sewing things. You put the lid back on and sulk. Another child enters the room and looks at the tin. You are asked what the child who has just entered the room will think is in the tin. A remarkable difference happens between the ages of three and five years old. A three-year-old will say 'sewing things'. They haven't yet learnt that the new person doesn't know what they do about the contents of the tin. Some four-year-olds and almost all five-year-olds, however, will say 'chocolates'. In that window of time, they have made a big leap in understanding that the experience and thinking of others is different to their own.

Three key things guide me in how I support Yvette to develop her theory of mind. Attachment is one. As discussed in Chapter 1, interaction and connection are integral to developing brains. They help with a child's early, superficial interpretation of what others experience as they start to learn about facial expressions, tones of voice and gestures. Another key element is exploring different perspectives in our play. I'll ask Yvette to show me how to make something for her, pretend I like something she doesn't (washing our hair) and ask what the toys we are playing with and the fictional characters in the books we are reading together are thinking. Pretend play is one of the best things we can do with kids to help them explore and learn about the world. The third factor is our parenting style. There is a huge cultural influence on parenting style, but one common finding in research is that warmth and authority play a big part in successfully helping our kids develop theory of mind and many other key social and emotional skills.[6]

If we look at these two distinct choices – 'tough love' versus prioritising connection – we can see four different styles:

- Being cold and strictly enforcing rules is called authoritarian parenting. It focuses on compliance and subsequent punishments, and it often challenges the relationship with the child, potentially impacting their self-esteem and prosocial development.
- Being cold but not having or enforcing rules is called neglectful parenting. It leaves kids on their own to figure out the world, and it has a devastating impact on brain development, emotional regulation and language skills.
- Being warm with our kids but not having or enforcing rules is called permissive parenting. This lack of guidance can lead to children having a really hard time when the expectations of school and peer relationships begin.

- Being warm and enforcing rules is called authoritative parenting. We have a lot of evidence saying it is the most effective style, because it promotes healthy self-esteem and development of goal setting, perspective taking and conflict resolution.

In authoritative parenting, the warmth of the relationship comes before the rules, and typically families discuss and make the rules together, so that kids hear an explanation for why the rule exists and can develop a shared understanding of its importance. As children get older, their autonomy and input to the rules can increase, building their sense of self and their role in the family unit. It is what all of us should aim for and it's closely tied with healthy development of theory of mind.

Let's return to twelve-year-old Omar. Over time, our assessment of Omar revealed that he was in fact very bright and, as his mother, Fatima, had said, he should be doing much better at school. We often see passing grades as good enough, even when children have a much higher potential. That said, grades aren't everything, and a child's level of social and emotional development is a much greater predictor of lifelong success.[7]

It is important that we harness a child's strengths when working with them to improve any gaps in their skills and development, and while trying to figure out how to help Omar, we were missing a big one. We discovered that Omar wasn't distracted in school, he just didn't care about it. He enjoyed being the class clown, but he was smart enough to avoid any significant consequences such as school suspensions by never crossing the line in his behaviour. He saw no reason to do more than just enough in his schoolwork. At home his mum had tried punishments, such as loss of internet privileges, but they seemed to have no impact. He would shrug his shoulders and tell his mum he didn't care. This had been going on for years now and was getting worse. Fatima had hoped that as he got older he would help around the house, but all he seemed to care about was himself. His younger siblings were observing his behaviour, and Fatima had started to notice their defiance emerging too.

While the early years are really important for the development of theory of mind, there is much we can do to help older kids with it too. Omar had successfully acquired the understanding that other people are different to us and have different perspectives, but hadn't yet achieved the next stage of understanding, which is that other people's thinking and reasoning might be different to our own. Just like everything in child development, we needed to show him this, not tell him.

Kids learn respect, reasoning and compromise through modelling more than anything else. I can simply ask Yvette to say sorry when she has done something wrong, but if I do that I'll miss the chance to show her why she should be saying sorry. The easiest way to teach this part is by saying sorry to her when I have done the wrong thing. It's important to demonstrate that we all make mistakes and this is okay. We then need to model the recovery between two people for them too.

On the rare occasions that Yvette has become overwhelmed and hit out physically, I try to think of theory of mind in my response: 'We don't hit, and no one should hit Yvette either.' The expectation isn't just about her actions, it's a common boundary that everyone needs to comply with. I explain why ('Because it hurts when people hit us and hurts when we hit them'), see if she has understood and then guide her to a more appropriate behaviour that is developmentally reasonable for her to achieve.

For older kids who are struggling with perspective and rules, we need to first show them that their experience is important. After validating this, we can then start to introduce how others see things. At the end of one appointment with Omar and Fatima, I handed them two pieces of paper with the numbers 1, 2 and 3 written down the side. I asked each of them to write down three things they would like from the other person. They needed to be specific, realistic and something that could happen at least once per week. At the next appointment, Omar walked in proudly with his list of three things: more video games, time with his friends and sleeping in on weekends. Fatima's three things were: Omar helping to prepare dinner, doing his homework and spending time with his little sister Yasmin.

Now was the fun part. I asked Fatima to read out what Omar had written and explain why he might want each one of them. She smiled at me, now working out the reason I'd done this. As she read them out, she non-judgementally explained why Omar had chosen each one. He enjoyed video games, loved his friends and usually stayed up late on the weekends, so he was tired in the mornings. Then it was Omar's turn. He found it harder than his mum, but he got there in the end. His mum had to feed five kids, so getting dinner on the table every night was tough. She always told him how smart he was, so the homework was to help him do better in school. Yasmin was only three years old and was really shy, but she really loved Omar and came out of her shell with him. It made sense that Fatima would want them to spend time together.

Fatima and I shared a quick smile. We made a plan that they would set these six goals for the next month and work on them together. In partnership, they would try each week to make sure they helped each other with these six things. Any time one of them was difficult, they would remind each other of the specific reason that goal was there. At the end of each week, they would talk about how they had gone. This is called reflective practice, and it is an important tool in parenting. All of us have different goals, but protecting time to reflect and talk about how we are going in this journey gives us a chance to decide what matters most to both ourselves and each other and how we can do better.

Relationship first

When children are struggling with certain aspects of development, such as understanding the perspective of others, it is important that we first reinforce the relationship. Then we can help the child to improve on that skill by setting small, specific and short-term goals. Choose a time to reflect on progress together and make the required adjustments. We need to make sure the goal is achieved frequently, ideally at least daily, and then immediately reinforced with celebration and praise.

> Finally, the most important aspect of helping our kids to improve at something is that we do it with them.

Over time, Fatima and Omar extended their goals and a strong partnership formed between them. They built sanctuaries together (watching movies Omar liked and learning recipes that Fatima knew Omar would use after he moved out) and Omar got to decide what his role in the family would be. Oldest children are sometimes forced into a parenting role that can be really destructive to their relationship with their younger siblings. While Omar wasn't forced to help out with Yasmin, Fatima did ask him to do so, which he tended to resist. But once he gained an understanding of her reasons for doing so, he was able to choose to do it and it became a positive experience that helped him to mature. In short, they had achieved mutual respect for each other's points of view.

The same strategy was used in his classroom too. Omar was given a leadership role that harnessed his strengths (confidence, intelligence and wit) and improved his relationship with his teacher. With time he understood the reason his teacher wanted more out of him in class, and his grades dramatically improved. He was still the class clown, but he understood when being a bit loud and silly was okay and when he needed to settle down and focus.

Any small opportunities you can find to show kids that they have a voice you value and want to understand can help them then learn that you have a voice too. It's important for them to learn that their own perspective and thoughts should be valued, but equally those of others should be valued too. That way they will be much more likely to succeed in their partnerships with others through their entire life.

Key lessons from Chapter 7:

- The relationship we have with our children must always come before and be more important than the rules we want to enforce. This is one of the most important aspects of building expectations and goals.
- Most of the effort of building the relationship occurs during times of calm. Showing children that they matter and have a voice gives us the best chance for the relationship to still hold during times of pressure and conflict.
- Children first learn about respect by receiving it from you and seeing you treat others with respect. That's how they learn to demonstrate these behaviours.

Strategies for parents:

- Help children to understand the reasons behind your rules and expectations, and ask them to explain why things might be important to them. This promotes shared understanding and respect for each other.
- As children get older, they should have more autonomy over their lives. Respecting them as individuals helps them to learn how to respect others, including us. This gradually increasing independence also gives them the best chance to thrive when they leave our care in adult life.
- If there is any concern about respect, then the first step is to connect and understand the child's perspective, then build the connection and prioritise their value over everything else. The relationship always comes before the rules.

8. Depression in kids does not present the same way as it does in adults.

Chapter 8

Depression

Depression in kids does not typically present the same way as it does for adults.[1] Low mood is much less frequent, and kids rarely tell you that they feel sad. Instead, they tend to show you, by pulling back from things they used to be interested in and struggling to focus. They get stuck in their thinking and often begin to make bad choices due to this clouding and indecision. For some teenagers, this tendency towards making poor choices coupled with a desire for social connection leads to them falling into antisocial peer groups. They can lose hope and become irritable, resulting in conflict with others, especially parents and teachers.

After anxiety, depression is the most common mental illness we see in children and teenagers, but it often gets missed.[2] Anxious kids usually show us through distress that something is wrong, whereas kids with depression often keep their struggles to themselves, because their illness disengages them from others. Given that they are the children at highest risk that we see in the clinic, and that 70 per cent of people with clinical depression will relapse (both adults and children), it is important that we know how to identify and respond to depression in the children and teens we support.[3]

If it wasn't for her family thinking she had ADHD, I'm not sure I would have ever met Alice. She was only fourteen years old when she first came to my clinic, but most would have thought she was much older. Her clothing, the way she spoke and how mature and bright she was regularly fooled people into thinking she was in her late teens. Even in that first appointment, I knew that people would be expecting too much of her, just like with many of the bright kids I meet in the clinic. I also sensed that she had been required to grow up too fast.

She came into my room with an older man named Nick, who I presumed was her father. Quickly Nick told me that he was Alice's uncle. He told me that he would be the one who would bring her to appointments and that I should speak to him if I needed anything, because she lived with his parents (Alice's grandparents), who didn't drive or talk on the phone. In fact, they rarely even left the house. Alice had been placed in their care about nine months earlier due to domestic violence in her parents' home, along with her younger brother, Alex, who was eleven years old. Nick was warm and likeable but very straight to the point. 'We are here for ADHD medication.'

'Okay, cool,' was my response. 'I prescribe that medication a fair bit, but we need to go through a few things before we get to talking about that. First, I need to learn about Alice.'

Nick responded with 'Fair enough, doc,' and we agreed to go over the whole story. He told me that Alice was exceptionally intelligent. In primary school she had skipped a year because the work was too easy for her. Despite being much younger than all of her classmates, she was still the top student in her class. Nick beamed with pride, telling me that she was the only smart one in the family. I asked him what other strengths she had. He told me she was really caring and good at looking after her younger brother. I sensed there was more to this, but also that Nick and Alice didn't feel comfortable discussing it yet. I also found out that she used to be really athletic, but for the past six months, she had stopped playing any of the sports she used to enjoy. She had also stopped seeing her friends.

Next we focused on difficulties. 'She can't sit still and is always daydreaming. Her grades are falling really low, and her teacher's worried. She says Alice is struggling to concentrate and is tired all of the time.'

Even though I already suspected more was going on with Alice, I can't tell you how many children I see with concerns about ADHD who are actually chronically sleep deprived. Think about those days, such as when you have to get an early morning flight, where you are short a few hours of sleep. You can't concentrate and are really agitated and forgetful. You don't have ADHD, though, but a huge sleep debt. Once you catch up on sleep, your focus and memory return to normal. So many kids aren't getting enough sleep, but they don't have the insight to realise that they are actually always tired. Given that ADHD medication can have a really negative impact on sleep, it's really important that we address this aspect before we even think about medication. It can be a hard issue to tackle, but often the best thing we can do for our kids, and ourselves, is to work on them getting better sleep.

Alice told me that she regularly took at least an hour to fall asleep and woke almost every night around 2 am, struggling to get back to sleep again. Finally she would wake early in the morning exhausted but unable to fall back asleep. Things were starting to add up in my head.

There are nine key clinical signs of depression. You need to have five of them for more than two weeks to meet diagnostic criteria, and one of those has to be either a low mood or the loss of interest in things you previously enjoyed.[4] In time, I would find out that Alice had a really low mood, but I had already heard about her loss of interest in school and extracurricular activities. She also had poor sleep, low energy, difficulty concentrating and 'psychomotor agitation', all of which are other symptoms of clinical depression.

Psychomotor agitation, also known as blunting, is often seen in kids with depression and can be helpful to be aware of when children don't have the language to say they are sad. It is a way that our nervous system shows us that it is struggling, either through restless activity as with Alice (for example, struggling to sit still, picking their skin or pulling at their clothing), or the opposite, with sluggish thinking, speech and movements. Other key features of depression are appetite or weight changes, feelings of worthlessness or guilt and thoughts about suicide.

Over time Alice would tell me that she was experiencing all of the symptoms and signs. Like many kids with mental illness, Alice's depression had developed during difficult times. Just like with all kids in crisis, I was at risk of focusing solely on her and missing the clues in her relationships and environment that would point me to the causes and strategies for recovery. As a developmental paediatrician, I have been trained to look beyond the patient in front of me and explore their family and broader community as integral influences both in the past and future.

Adverse childhood experiences can lead to developmental trauma in children. Many people will know about abuse and neglect, but household dysfunction is also a significant contributor to issues with development and mental health. Parental conflict, substance abuse, mental illness and violence within families has a devastating impact on child development, because the challenge to the child's safety and security stunts their brain growth and increases the risk of mental illness. These experiences echo through their thoughts, further traumatising them even when the danger has gone. This developmental trauma can easily be incorrectly diagnosed as conditions such as ADHD, autism and anxiety, because children who have experienced hostile environments and relationships often show signs of difficulty in their behaviour.

In some kids we may think isolated clinical anxiety is the cause of their difficulties, but they may have experienced significant events and the fear of them was not a mental illness, but a reasonable response. For other children, their coping mechanisms might involve self-isolation and avoidance, impacting their relationships in a way that may seem like autism. In others still, poor concentration and hyper vigilance can seem like the attention and hyperactivity seen in ADHD, as with Alice. A complicating factor is that children with these conditions are also at a greater risk of developmental trauma, as their needs exceed the capacity of their caregivers.[5] They are also at risk of carrying these experiences through into their own parenting journey, continuing the cycle of multigenerational trauma. Catching issues like developmental trauma and mental illness in these kids early, caring for them and guiding them through these tough journeys creates healthier communities for generations to come.

As kids get older, we try to give them more control over the care they receive in our clinic, whereas young kids often need adults to be their voice. Alice was old enough that she didn't need Nick to be with her at appointments, and so a lot of our time together was spent with just the two of us. I learnt so much about her and from her in those moments.

Following assessment, we all agreed that Alice did not have ADHD, but she did need treatment for depression. There are two main approaches to this, both applicable to Alice's situation. The first involved decreasing her stress. I had learnt that her grandparents were very strict. After school, Alice had to complete a list of chores and homework that meant she had no free time. Even if she wanted to, there was no opportunity to engage with her friends. Her grandparents also didn't allow her to have any access to technology, limiting her social connection opportunities even further. Besides leaving the house for school, Alice had been told she had to see her parents in supervised visits. Having gone through these as a little kid, I understood how awful they could be. Having a stranger present while you try to have quality time with a family member is a pretty horrible experience for all involved. Nick told me Alice was often really shut down after these visits and was even less talkative than usual. First, we needed to remove as much stress as possible for Alice and increase her support. The second approach involved individual therapy. Alice started seeing an amazing psychologist I worked with called Jess, who I knew would help to guide her through these tough times.

Like lots of children with depression, Alice was stuck. Young people often become stuck because of three mistakes their brain makes about their situation. First, they think everything is their fault: everything negative is because of them, whereas anything positive is due to luck, or is diminished in some other way. Second, they think the negative experience will permeate through every part of their life: all of their relationships will fall apart, everyone will realise they are worthless and the failure they are experiencing in one area will eventually spread to all the others. Finally, they think it is permanent: the feeling of hopelessness is so overwhelming that it takes away any ability to see life on the other side of it.

Loss of hope can be so devastating that a person doesn't want to live anymore. I have an intimate knowledge of this debilitating mental illness. I was clinically depressed, saw no reason to live and at times didn't really want to. It was a period in my adult life that was by far the most difficult I've ever gone through, and these feelings completely overwhelmed me for over a year. This experience did, however, help me to relate to children with depression and gave me an instinctive ability to create safe and open spaces for kids to share their feelings. It also made me all the more determined to protect my own kids from this illness as much as it's possible to, especially since my history places them at higher risk.

Self-harm and what to do

Supporting a child who is self-harming can be a traumatising experience. Research indicates that 10–20 per cent of teenagers have self-harmed, highlighting the fact that many of the children we care for will have to face this harrowing experience.[6]

There are many reasons that individuals self-harm, including underlying mental illness, social isolation, low self-esteem, bullying, family dysfunction or trauma. It can be a coping mechanism for dealing with overwhelming emotions such as anger, sadness, rejection or stress. It may be a distraction technique to take the focus off other, more distressing aspects of life. For some it can be a way to feel in control when so much feels out of control, or it may be a way to feel something when they feel numb. Others tell us that it is a form of self-punishment for a failure in their lives. In all cases it should be seen as a signal that someone needs our support.

When responding to self-harm, try as much as possible to remain calm. An approach of empathy and acknowledgement can help show the person who is struggling that we care. Our role should be to prioritise healing using simple first aid principles, along with a calm voice and phrases such as 'I can see that you're hurt. How can I help?'

Our aim is to listen non-judgementally. We should not ask for an explanation, because many children will not know why they are self-harming. It also challenges the role of unconditional support that we're striving for. If the child does tell you why they are harming themselves, we should also try not to dismiss the experience, as it is very real for the child. Our goal in these moments is safety and connection.

Finally, all families struggling with this should seek urgent support from health services. This is not something you should have to manage alone.

At the end of our third appointment together I asked Alice if there was anything else she would like to say. She hesitated and then said, 'No'. I told her that was fine but if it was okay with her, I'd like to just sit with her for a bit longer in case something came up. She didn't reply but she stayed seated. Slowly tears started rolling down her face. I didn't say anything and just handed her a tissue. Within a couple of minutes, she was sobbing. I resisted the urge to say, 'It's okay' and just kept sitting with her. When the big flood of tears had finally passed, I told her that I could see her pain, that we could sit there as long as needed and that she didn't need to talk. Then I told her that what she was experiencing was not her fault and that it wasn't fair. I spoke about it being an illness, just like asthma, and told her that there were so many things we could do to treat it. I told her that I would see her in the clinic for as long as needed until what she was feeling was gone. Then I asked one of the hardest questions we ever ask: 'Have you ever wanted to die?' Alice stared right at me and subtly nodded.

Suicidal ideation and what to do

There is a myth that asking people about suicide might put that idea in their minds. In truth, most kids who are experiencing suicidal ideation have been dealing with it alone long before anyone mentions it to them.[7] Given that it is the highest cause of death in people aged 15–45, it is important that we get better at talking about it as soon as possible. For anyone worried about this in your kids, it is important that you feel comfortable to ask about it. Tell them you are worried about them, and that you care and want to help. It is important to ensure you stay calm and non-judgemental when you ask, as this helps to make kids feel safe. Don't ask them to explain why they feel the way they do, as often they can't tell you. You should also try to avoid making them feel guilty, as this only isolates them further. And you should never promise to keep it a secret. Instead, you should promise to do whatever you can to help.

Suicide is very different to self-harm, but both are a sign of kids who are extremely overwhelmed and often a cry for help. Children experiencing either suicidal ideation or self-harm always need professional support. No caregiver or professional without training should try to support these kids alone.

Keeping kids safe in these circumstances can often mean staying with them until that professional help comes. One thing we can ask is what has helped them feel better before. For Alice, those things were out of reach at this time, but we needed to find a way to bring them back into her life. She needed a break from the weight of her chores, her homework and the supervised visits with her parents. I found out that their own mental health was also deteriorating and they were in their own crisis, which clinicians were now treating. It was important for us to protect Alice from seeing them in mental turmoil, as I knew this would give them the best chance at a healthy relationship in the future. We also needed to help Alice see her friends. Nick agreed to take some time off work to do this. This began with small social opportunities with just one other teenager, whose parents were very caring. Finding non-parental adults who genuinely care about your child and allowing them to spend time together is one of the most protective things you can do. It increases their self-esteem in times of calm and provides an additional safety net when things become tough. Having multiple people you can turn to for support and guidance is something all of us should be striving for.

We also worked on Alice's sleep. The waking overnight was a symptom of her depression and would take time to improve, but I could help her with the difficulty falling asleep right away. We decided that Alice would only go into her bedroom when she was tired. She needed to read and study in another room, because she was lying for hours on her bed with a book in hand, ruminating and catastrophising. This meant she was subconsciously linking her bed and her negative thought patterns, affecting her sleep. By separating the two, we saw within a couple of weeks that she was falling asleep more quickly.

Now that she had a healthy association with her bed and sleep, we slowly brought her bedtime forward to give her a longer sleep period. This technique is called bedtime fading, and it is incredibly effective – maybe even better than medication! – if done correctly. I myself know that personally, as my sleep hygiene is terrible. I am often up late at night writing about what others should do that I can't do myself.

In moderate to severe cases of depression, there is evidence that using a combination of therapy and medication is helpful to re-establish healthy thoughts and behaviours.[8] We decided to use this approach with Alice. The medication is the easy bit – it helps to increase firing of the parts of the brain that improve our mood. While this is helpful, it is rarely enough on its own, because of a common saying about medication for children: pills don't teach skills.

The skills that people with depression generally need to focus on are how to manage negative thoughts. Alice had spent so long interpreting the world as cold, hostile and hopeless that it became her natural thinking pattern. In many ways, this attitude was justified, based on her previous experiences of household dysfunction. Even though we had improved her environment and introduced some protective factors like getting more sleep and seeing her friends, we now needed to help her relearn ways of interpreting the world. Alice explained to me that she didn't want to try at school anymore because she might not be as smart as everyone thought she was. This is not unusual with smart children, as people tend to focus on their strengths, which can make them even more vulnerable to falling apart. They can become so dependent upon this strength that any risk of failing in it challenges their entire identity. She also told me she felt like everything that happened between her parents was her fault, which is common among children who have experienced developmental trauma.

The team of adults in Alice's corner, including me, Nick, psychologist Jess and Alice's teachers, all supported her in introducing different interpretations of the world. Having these safe relationships allowed Alice to become comfortable sharing her negative thoughts, and with time, she learnt how to gently challenge them. 'I'll fail at the test' could be acknowledged but responded to with 'What else might happen?' 'No one wants me around' could be answered with specific examples of others who valued her company. Using open questions, silence when you sense a child has something on their mind, validation, empathy and gentle optimism can all help a child to feel safe enough to tell you about their inner turmoil.

This type of supportive reinforcement, free of pressure, can help build healthier ways for kids to interpret the world. A single traumatic event can scar us mentally and it takes repeated, consistent and predictable positive experiences to heal those wounds. With Yvette, I try to build her healthy thinking at a very basic level. I try to teach her about emotions through play, my own experiences and helping her put words around her own feelings. I try to validate all her emotions and slowly introduce the difference between how she is feeling and how she is acting. Being sad sometimes is normal, and expecting support when you are feeling this way should be normal too. At two and a half, Yvette can name sadness in books and provide basic ideas for what might help that character. Her ideas are often based on what would make her feel better rather than the character, but that's okay at this stage in her development. With time I will help teach her that what others need when sad can be different to what she needs.

It is also important that I acknowledge Yvette's positive emotions and the activities that have led to them. Often as parents we get so caught up in the negative emotions in our kids that we don't give the attention or energy to their antidote. Every child is different, but positive routines, exercise, creativity and calming activities help to build healthy experiences and expectations of the world. When a child is depressed, small, supported steps towards these activities help to build their ability to eventually turn to them on their own when their mood is low.

In Alice's case, we found her mood improved when she started to engage socially and slowly stepped back into activities she used to enjoy. At first she went to watch netball. Then, after a month, she decided she was happy to fill in when they needed an extra player. Soon after that she was playing full games each week. Her grandparents were persuaded to let her have access to social media to stay in touch with her friends and explore some of her creative pursuits. Social media gets blamed for so much of the mental illness in the world these days, but it's really how we use it that matters. I've seen many children use it as a stepping stone to reconnect with their peers and find their people, interests and purpose.

I don't see Alice in the clinic anymore these days. I know she's in safe hands with her amazing psychologist, teachers and uncle. The last I heard she was going to therapy monthly, no longer needed medication and was back succeeding at school socially and academically. She was seeing her parents but still living with her grandparents. Her little brother was back living with their mum and dad, but it was too soon for Alice. Often the pace of recovery we want kids to go at is not possible for them. As supports, we must remember that we are cheerleaders, not pacesetters. All that matters is that the children we support move forward and that when they look around, they see us by their side helping them keep going. Alice will always have a path back to me if she ever needs it, as there is nothing better in the world than cheering for the kids who are in our lives.

Key lessons from Chapter 8:

- Depression in children looks different to depression in adults. It can be really difficult for kids to realise and tell us they feel sad. Often it presents with agitation and shutting down, but self-isolation can worsen their mental health and place them at greater risk of very serious consequences such as self-harm and suicide.
- Other signs of depression are the loss of interest in a child's usual activities, changes in appetite or weight, sleep difficulties, fatigue, feeling worthless, excessive guilt, poor concentration, indecision and thoughts of suicide. Their feelings of worthlessness, hopelessness and guilt cause them to become stuck in the belief that things will always be this way no matter what they do.
- All children need to have safe spaces and opportunities to talk about negative feelings. We need to address those feelings and help children develop healthy beliefs and thought processes to challenge them. In addition, we need to support healthy behaviours such as sleep, exercise and positive relationships as much as possible in all children.

Strategies for parents:

- If you are concerned that your child is feeling low, shutting down or easily agitated, then it is important to think about what might be going on for them and their overall functioning. Speaking to key people at school and others in their life can help to gain an understanding of how they are going when not in your care.
- Many children who are depressed show us this through changes in other parts of their life. Focusing on those areas can improve their mood. Children with poor sleep benefit from focusing on improving this, just as kids with deteriorating concentration, social engagement or self-talk need support here too.
- When talking to kids who are sad or low, it is essential that they don't feel judged or that it is their fault. These children need validation and empathy. Parents and other professionals should also seek specialist support from experts such as a developmental paediatrician, psychologist or psychiatrist early, as often this is required to restore their mood.

9. There's no such thing as a bad kid.

Chapter 9

'Bad' kids

Every child has unique needs. In many cases these needs can be met by parents and teachers without much cause for extra support from doctors and other professionals, but in some cases, children have higher needs. While a diagnosis such as autism or ADHD can be helpful as a guide for providing support, we need to be aware of the risk that a label will start to define a child. It's unfortunately all too easy to focus on the diagnosis or label, and lose sight of their individual identity. When seeking a diagnosis, it's important to consider if the benefit will outweigh the risk.

In my experience there are two diagnoses where the benefit never comes close to the risk: Oppositional Defiant Disorder (ODD) and Conduct Disorder (CD). These are two diagnoses that I have never made and I hope I never have to.

I've met hundreds of children who have been given these labels before coming to our clinic and all of them were defined by that label. ODD and CD can be thought of as a sequence.

ODD usually comes before CD and is often diagnosed in younger primary school kids.[1] CD is diagnosed at an older age, often late in primary school and during secondary school. Both disorders include antisocial behaviour that has a significant negative impact on others. Often these children have severe behavioural difficulties, are hostile towards authority figures and frequently become violent and damage property.

Many of these children have been told they are 'naughty' or 'bad' since they were toddlers. With time they get comfortable with this narrative and may even believe it – if it's all they've known, this story becomes their only story as they are blamed for household conflict and classroom chaos. If you're in the throes of trying to deal with challenging behaviour on an ongoing basis, it's easy to forget that these are just kids, and not some sinister force waking up each morning with a plan of misery and destruction. But these stories are often the biggest problem, as I truly believe that we become what people tell us we are.

A diagnosis of ODD or CD is only a description of symptoms and gives no insight into the underlying cause. Often the cause is due to these children having emotional, social or intellectual difficulties that result in them being caught up in a cycle of failure and negative experiences. As we learnt in Chapter 1, a child's sensitive temperament can result in insecure attachment and difficulty regulating their emotions. Conflict and rejection become the norm for these kids, which has a significant impact on their relationships, self-esteem and mental health. They are at a huge risk of becoming isolated from the community, which in turn increases the risk of them becoming antisocial adults with addiction, mental illness and criminal behaviours, further burdening them and those around them.[2] All of the adults trapped in these situations were once children who most likely tried to succeed but failed. It is everyone in the community's role to help change the trajectory of these kids, as all of us benefit from the outcomes of doing so. If not, we will feel the ongoing fracturing of our society, as children who are left behind become adults who are scarred from their journey.

I was one of the fortunate few 'bad' kids whose trajectory was changed. As a child, I was repeatedly told I'd never amount to anything. I kept hearing it in my teenage years and even my early twenties. Becoming a doctor changed that, as if somehow I had discovered a part of me that wasn't there before. Many of my teachers were happy to see me go when I was kicked out of high school. I'd left such an impression that no other school in the area wanted me either. My mum had no idea what was going on. She was working so much in her full-time job and waitressing after hours that I was getting away with frequently skipping school, getting in trouble when I did go and drinking regularly. For years I had been participating in antisocial behaviours, and I cringe at the damage I caused and the risks I took as a teenager. I was lost and struggling with the adversity that I and many of my friends had grown up with. We knew no better and were seeking thrills and some kind of identity for ourselves. I think we were also looking for connection and not finding it in the more traditional places like home, school and sports.

I was seen as a bad kid by adults and my peers, and I settled in comfortably to that story. If it wasn't for a school principal called Brian, I'm not sure what would have happened to me. I'd been rejected from half-a-dozen schools and this was the last one. Brian gave me a chance when no other principal would. He and the school helped break the cycle of hostility that would go on to change my story. There was no conflict with teachers. I was seen as a valued member of the classroom from day one. If I didn't submit an assignment, that was my choice. I was offered support, but the grade was my consequence, nothing else. If I didn't submit anything, my value wasn't reduced. It was the opposite to what I had experienced in all the previous years of secondary education. Now I, in turn, try to change the story of others.

Like all of us who are parents, my own childhood informs how I guide my children. There is no bigger influence on how we parent.[3] Yvette, like all toddlers, has moments of very challenging behaviour. Given her generally easygoing temperament, they don't happen too frequently and she usually settles quickly. She and Charlie are relatively easy to parent, and if I didn't know better due to my profession, I would be vulnerable to some pretty high levels of false confidence, just like when I thought I had it in the bag the first night we brought her home from hospital.

While Yvette is in no way at risk of a diagnosis of ODD or CD, I want to do everything I can to keep it that way. I am constantly trying to improve how I respond to her, and I try to be very proactive in how I contribute to her story. Everything we give attention to, we reinforce, so when Yvette decides to throw her dinner onto the floor, I have to decide if this is something I want to give attention to. If it is, I had better be ready to meet her needs in that moment and help her learn a better way to engage with us and her food at meal times. If I don't have that in me and there is no risk in the behaviour, I should simply ignore it and give attention to something else, such as how good she is at using her Peter Rabbit spoon.

Kids are wired to engage with their environment. They often don't care about right or wrong, because receiving attention is way more important to them. So much of their behaviour is about seeking connection. I am constantly looking for specific things to praise Yvette for, be it helping us to feed our dog, Melfi, rocking Charlie when he's upset or sharing in her play. There are constantly opportunities to bring a positive narrative into her story.

I hope that I never challenge who Yvette is or speak of her in a negative way, even if her behaviour is difficult. I want to make sure I separate the things she does from her identity. I also try my hardest not to battle with her, because I want to limit conflict between us as much as possible. At the moment, this is most difficult in the evenings. Even though she is clearly tired, she fights going to bed every single night. Once the toothbrush comes out, the chase begins. She's off and running, refusing to take the last step before getting into bed.

If I'm honest, at times I get pretty agitated when this happens. Desperate to get back to work or finish some chores or spend time with Annaliese and somehow still get enough sleep, I can feel my heart rate rising as I try to convince Yvette to come and brush her teeth and get into bed. It's in these moments, though, that we learn to work with our kids, not against them. It adds a few extra minutes to the process, but

I've learnt that a playful approach often works. A quick lap of chasing her or the toothbrush coming alive and asking nicely to clean her teeth can usually steer her towards brushing her teeth with minimal distress. I stuff this up almost as much as I succeed at it and it sometimes ends with her tears (thankfully not mine, usually!). Luckily, I have another chance to get better at it the next night.

While this is a very small example of a challenging moment in my life as a parent, far smaller than the situations I see coming up in the clinic, it does highlight the importance of remembering that the responsibility to improve should sit with us, not the children we are supporting. We need to change our approach to meet the needs of our kids and help them through these moments, building their confidence and knowledge that we love them no matter what.

With kids who are really out of control, we often unintentionally reinforce their unwanted behaviour. When they sense rejection or conflict, their fight response quickly kicks in. Instead of staying in the discomfort of the unknown, they seek out the predictable outcome and lash out. This is especially true for any children with sensitivity to negative emotions, such as those who have experienced trauma. For them, predictable means safe. So, the battle begins. We issue threats of punishments and consequences, which the child matches with the risk of escalation in their behaviour. One of two things will happen. Either our threats work and the child is punished, or our threats don't work and the child wins through intimidation or increasing concerns of safety. Neither outcome is good, because the successful strategy – either threats or escalation – for ending the conflict has been reinforced, and whoever 'won' is more likely to use this move in future conflict.

In truth, though, there are no winners in that fight. No parent enjoys making threats, let alone having to follow through on them, and the child is not getting what they want either, even if it might seem like it on the surface. This pattern is called the coercive cycle, and it increases negative behaviours in children and threatens the relationship.[4]

So what would be a better alternative? In moments of emotional difficulty, we need to first regulate ourselves, connect with the child and then guide them to healthier and more appropriate behaviours. There is always a reason that the child is struggling, and a big part of improving things is finding that reason and addressing it. It might be developmental trauma, anxiety or a learning difficulty, or numerous other things, but most things can be improved in partnership with everyone supporting the child.

The other part of the solution is changing their story. We need to break the pattern, and that starts with telling a new story.

Jayden was sixteen years old when he was first sent to see me by child protection. It's not uncommon for me to meet kids this way, and it's one of the greatest opportunities I get to help a child and make a difference in their life. He was sitting on his own in the waiting room when I went out to meet him. He was small for his age and had on an oversized black hoodie with the hood up over large headphones. He didn't hear me call his name, but I walked over. He looked at me, pulled his hood down and took his headphones off, revealing an NBA cap and a thick silver chain around his neck. I already knew Jayden was going to be fun to get to know.

I introduced myself and directed Jayden to my room. For a second he didn't move, and I thought he might tell me to get stuffed. Fair enough, I guess – no one wants to be forced to see a specialist because of how much trouble they're getting in. But he got up and followed me, swaggering down the corridor to show me very early on that things were going to go at his pace. In my office he slumped into the chair and I sat down opposite him. I quickly noticed that I was unintentionally sitting the same way as him, already trying to connect with him before we had even started the appointment. Jayden brought that out in me a lot actually. I mirrored his body language and found myself reverting to the slang of my days working in factories driving forklifts. Like many social interactions, working in the clinic was a dance and I wanted to match Jayden's moves to see where he would take me.

That first appointment was just with Jayden and me. We actually didn't talk about anything to do with why he was there. When I first asked how I could help, he just shrugged. He had been brought in by a social worker who had gone to get a coffee in the hospital cafe while we talked, but Jayden had just met him that morning when he picked him up for the appointment, so they hadn't had much of a chance to talk yet. So Jayden and I just talked. It took a while to find a connection, but once I found out he liked skateboarding, I knew I had a way in. I have a huge scar on my right wrist from a severe skateboarding injury. It gets me a lot of credibility with kids like Jayden who think I'm just another boring adult. We also connected over video games, another hobby I tell Annaliese I need to keep up for my clinical work. At the end of that first appointment, I told Jayden that I thought I could make things better for him. He looked at me and said he wasn't sure. I asked if he could just give me a chance and come back. He said, 'Yeah, fair enough. It gets me out of school at least.' Fair point, I guess.

Jayden lived with his grandmother, Gwen, who I met at a later appointment. She was a phenomenal woman who believed in Jayden when everyone else had given up on him. She had taken him in years ago when his dad went to prison. No one had any idea where his mum was, but Gwen thought that was for the best. Jayden had been kicked out of three schools, and his current school was his final chance. I knew this school well, as it was often the saving step for many kids who were going off the deep end. Jayden didn't like the place, but he said it was better than the others. He'd tried to burn down the previous school. Gwen told me that after that happened, the fire department sent a guy around to teach Jayden about fire safety. It didn't go well. Jayden and the guy got into a heated argument and Gwen had to separate them and ask the man to leave. She never heard from the fire department after that.

I'm not sure what the plan was in sending someone to talk to Jayden about fire safety, but I think there were probably more pressing issues at hand. His destructive behaviour was a symptom, rather than the underlying problem. When he was younger he had seen another developmental paediatrician who had diagnosed him with oppositional defiant disorder and then conduct disorder. I'm sure that specialist tried to get to the cause of those behaviours, but I don't think they'd had much success, given how things were going for Jayden.

Jayden confided in me that he'd started carrying around a knife, because he'd been attacked at the train station about a month ago. He was so wired for threats that he saw them everywhere. His developmental trauma was ongoing, as he was still placing himself in risky situations without the skills needed to navigate them. He was drinking and using drugs with other kids who had been kicked out of school. No one had supported Jayden to learn to manage risks safely, so he didn't know how to handle the risks he was being exposed to. He needed a guide.

Learning about risks

We tend to think of risk as being something teenagers learn, and so we form a plan to one day have a chat with our future teens about drugs, sex and other risky behaviours. But children learn about risk in their very early years. As toddlers have a burst of development in the motor and language parts of their brain, they become little adventurers, and this is when they start to learn about risk. Our role is to help our kids learn about risk from this early stage, not shield them from it completely. 'Safe enough, not as safe as possible' is a helpful mantra. By being overly cautious, we limit their growth in learning to navigate risk on their own.

Jayden also needed a different story. Currently he was on a one-way road to a pretty bad place. I asked him about his future, and he seemed fairly resigned, saying, 'I'll probably get kicked out of school and sell drugs.' He saw no healthy options. With time, I got to know him and saw that he had so many strengths. He was really brave, and he had a strong sense of social justice. He just couldn't see how his own behaviour was in conflict with that at times. He cared about other people but had little ability to trust them. It was much safer to assume all of those relationships were conditional, so he might as well destroy them before people abandoned him first.

I told Jayden often that he was better than the current story about him. It took a long time to convince him of that though, and in truth, it wasn't me who pulled it off. It rarely is, as I play such a small role in these kids' lives, really. They see me for half an hour every month or so, in the foreign world of a consultation room, far away from the rest of their world. The person who sparked the change in Jayden was a guy in his twenties called Ali, who worked for a youth mentoring program. I'd heard about the program and helped get Jayden in. He was reluctant at first, but I asked him to do me a favour and give it a try. Well, Ali nailed it. Within a couple of months of them being paired up and hanging out weekly, Ali was the authority on everything. Any suggestions I made to Jayden needed to be discussed with Ali first, and appointments with me needed to be moved if they ever clashed with Ali. They would hang out and have fun together. I got to know Ali too, and I could see the magic in what he was doing. While he was helping Jayden learn how to navigate his emotions and manage risks, he was also helping to change his story. Even though Ali was getting paid to spend time with Jayden, I could tell he really cared about him. With time, Jayden saw that too.

One day Jayden came to the clinic with his dad, Trent. I didn't know much about him, but I'd had no idea he had been released. Jayden was so excited to introduce me to him. He was a pretty tough guy. 'Hey, doc. Jayden tells me you're a Frankston boy?' Coincidentally, Trent had grown up in the same town I had, a rough outer suburb of Melbourne known back then for its housing estates, its low employment and its high crime rates. I'd actually had no idea of this reputation growing up. I thought it was a great place as it had playgrounds, a beach and a good skatepark. It was only when I moved out to go to medical school that I found out about its reputation. I wanted to fit in so much with the private school students in my class that for the first year I lied about where I was from. When my mum found out, she really scolded me. She worked at the Frankston city council and was proud of her community. It was a positive part of her story, and now I understand that it is for me too. My background allows me to connect with others like Trent, giving me the best chance to build a partnership with them.

I noticed a change in Jayden during that appointment with his dad. When I asked him how things had been, he told me how happy he was to be hanging out with his father. Trent was staying at one of his mate's houses until he got a place of his own. Jayden was staying there too. I asked what Gwen thought, and Trent replied, 'She's too strict with him, so he's better off with me. All she wants him to do is go to school and do homework. Jayden doesn't need that stuff. He's already lasted longer than I did at school, and one of my mates will find him a job in construction anyway'.

Jayden smiled and nodded at me when his dad said this, and I learnt that Jayden had stopped attending school since his dad got out of prison, and he had also missed a couple of catch-ups with Ali. 'It's fine,' he told me.

I noted that Jayden's knuckles were bruised and bloodied, and asked what had happened. Jayden looked at his dad and smiled. 'Nothing he couldn't handle,' Trent said with pride.

I could see all the progress Jayden had made slipping away in front of me. I asked him if I could chat to his dad alone. Jayden agreed and went down the corridor to the waiting room. As I closed the door behind him, I questioned whether what I was doing was right. I wouldn't normally risk the relationship with a parent at the first appointment, but I was really worried I wasn't going to see Jayden at the clinic again. I sat down and faced Trent. 'It's so amazing to see how happy you make Jayden. He really looks up to you'. Trent smiled and agreed. 'He's a good kid, you know, but I'm really worried about him,' I continued. Trent shot me back a puzzled frown. 'Over the last six months he's made such amazing progress. He's been doing so well at school, he's learning so much from Ali and staying off drugs.'

Trent didn't seem that impressed. I told him that I thought Jayden is actually a really sensitive, brave and compassionate kid. 'I think he looks up to you and wants to impress you so much that he is trying to be like you. I know you've had a tough time, but I'm not sure he's as tough as you. He might not be able to handle the same road without it hurting him.' I spoke about how I could see so many options for Jayden if he stayed in school, opportunities for him to take advantage of how great he was. I shared my own story and the options I'd been given. Trent sat there listening, not giving me any sign of what he thought, but I could tell he was taking it in. 'I can see how much you love him and that you want the best for him. He idolises you so much that with your help, I think he has a really bright future ahead of him.'

I had no idea if I'd crossed a line or not. I'd hoped that by highlighting their relationship and the potential of his influence over Jayden, I hadn't challenged Trent as a parent. 'Let me think about it, mate,' was the only response I got. We both walked out to the waiting room together so I could say goodbye to Jayden. Time would tell if I had pulled it off or not.

I never saw Trent again after that meeting, but Jayden did come back. He was a bit pissed off, because his dad had said he needed to go back to living with Gwen – something about his mate needing the space. But I was pleased to see Jayden was back at school and hanging out with Ali again. He was still drinking with his mates, but he told me he was going easy on the other stuff. He was still getting to see his dad and wished he was still living with him, as Gwen was always hassling him about getting up for school and homework.

He was reluctantly doing it, though, and his school told me that he was back succeeding there again.

The most recent appointment I had with Jayden was just before the school holidays. I asked him what he was looking forward to over the break. He told me he had just got a job in a supermarket, stacking shelves, thanks to one of the teachers at his school. He wanted to save up so he could buy a car. He had been learning to drive with Gwen, and in a year he would be able to go for his licence. He wanted to drive up the east coast of Australia but had decided to finish school first. He wasn't sure what he wanted to do once he was done, but he was happy for me to keep talking to him about his options. Jayden is one of the many teens that I am still working with and will be sad to say goodbye to one day. He is a brilliant example of how the best way to shake a negative story is to replace it with a positive one.

Key lessons from Chapter 9:

- The story around a child can have a huge influence on who they become. Many children with developmental and mental health difficulties can be really challenging to support. These challenging interactions become the norm and the child gets comfortable with conflict and opposition. In giving attention to this conflict, we reinforce it and its role in defining the child.
- Kids care more about predictability than pleasing others. Children repeat behaviours that they know the outcome of, such as lashing out at home or school. The consequence of lashing out ends the difficult situation for everyone, unintentionally increasing the chance it will happen again.
- Any time a child is acting out, we need to decide if we have the capacity to support them. If we don't, then safety is all that matters. If we do, then our role is to guide them to what we want them to be doing. Through calm, connection and understanding, we can team up with the child to help them succeed.

Strategies for parents:

- Try as hard as you can to always be on the same side as your child and build a positive narrative around them. When things are tough, talk about how we know that as a team we can do better.
- Every child and teenager needs predictability and success. Finding small opportunities frequently to succeed at things means that they come to see themselves as someone worthy of praise during effort and support during struggles.
- In really difficult scenarios we must remember that as adults we have greater abilities and capacity to find the path through. If we are finding it overwhelming, you can guarantee that deep down, the child is too. We must be kind and gentle with ourselves and the child we are supporting.

10. Your mental health is important too.

Chapter 10

You

By far the most difficult role I have in the clinic is addressing the mental health needs of parents. To help a family, it's essential for me to form a partnership with them. In all of my years of clinical practice, the most common reason I have failed to establish a partnership has been when parental mental illness was too great a barrier for me to overcome.

In every stage of parenting, we are vulnerable to being overwhelmed by stress when the demands placed upon us exceed our capacity. Supporting children with developmental and mental health concerns places a huge mental load on parents. Parenting is challenging enough without the additional hurdle of navigating emotional and behavioural difficulties in your child. This stress, especially when it is prolonged, can challenge healthy attachment and lead to mental illness in us, too.

Unfortunately, parents rarely prioritise their own mental health. They will tell me that their child's needs matter more or that there isn't anything to worry about, and they don't ask for support. Sometimes they say, 'Once my child is better, I will be too.' The reality, however, is that addressing the parents' mental health is often the first step to helping their child, and without looking at that, my ability to help is drastically limited.

I know this from personal experience – my own mental health influences my parenting so much. I believe that we are individuals first, partners next (if we are in a relationship) and parents third. Many of the parents I meet in the clinic disagree with that view. They see themselves as parents first. I'm not a fan of the saying 'You need to put your own oxygen mask on first', because the plane crash analogy only really relates to moments of chaos, but in order to be the best parent we can, we must at times prioritise our own mental health. We build our own capacity and wellbeing by constantly working at it, not only addressing it when the plane hits turbulence. By then it is often too late.

Genetics and mental health

Genetic risk means that many of the children I meet have a family history of developmental and mental health concerns. Parents are often unaware of this and first discover their own diagnosis of conditions such as anxiety or depression by participating in our assessment of their child.

Looking after our own mental health fuels our ability to meet our family's needs. Being stressed, sleep deprived and angry is one sure way to make life harder for ourselves. It's also a sure way to fail to model emotions well. By that I don't mean we should always be modelling emotions perfectly. We should not aim for perfect, firstly because it's impossible and secondly because it risks teaching our kids that perfection is the goal. By showing kids that we also fail at controlling our emotions, we allow them to accept that they will too. Occasionally losing our temper and yelling or making threats of punishment gives us the chance to model the most important part, the recovery.

By showing what happens after we lose our temper or become emotionally unregulated, we help our kids to learn what their own strategies might be when they feel stressed and overwhelmed. Yvette sees me stressed frequently, but I try to acknowledge it, use words to describe what I'm feeling and then make sure she can see my process for dealing with it. Whether it's calming myself down by focusing on my breathing, asking for support from Annaliese or going for a run, I want her to see the effort I make to deal with difficult emotions, in the hope that it helps her navigate those pathways to recovery too.

If you're struggling with your child's behavioural difficulties, addressing your own mental health is possibly the best thing you can do. Accessing the support of a therapist is beneficial, if it's within your means. The times I've seen a therapist have been such positive experiences and helped me improve my mental health, and I've witnessed these positive effects in the parents I meet in the clinic, too. We all need people in our lives who support us, but there is something unique about seeing a mental health professional with whom you can safely discuss your darkest fears, without feeling guilty, selfish or that you are risking the other relationships in your life.

I often worry that many young children only hear about negative emotions when they are overwhelmed, leading to shame about these feelings and thinking they must always be happy, grateful or content. I think we do that to ourselves too, carrying that experience as children into our adult lives and then through to our parenting approach.

Sadly, many adults don't feel comfortable seeking out support, either because they think they don't need it or because they see it as a sign of personal weakness. We don't do that with diseases like cancer or issues like allergies, so I'm not sure why we do it with mental illness. My own mental illness was no more my fault than my hayfever or asthma, and it required treatment just as they did. The stigma of mental illness is so destructive to our communities, and it's something I always make a point to normalise at every opportunity I get.

Evidence tells us that behavioural difficulties in children are often linked to reactive and harsh parenting approaches.[1] By building the ability of parents to be calm, warm and consistent, we create a pathway for behaviours to improve, which in turn further addresses the mental health of the parent. The negative cycle can be turned into a positive one, but usually it requires that the parent makes the first step.

Asking for help

If you're finding yourself stuck in supporting a child, then reaching out for help is a really important but difficult step to take. We worry that we shouldn't need to ask for help, but not asking often leads to things getting worse. Trusted individuals in our community are often the best people to go to first. Your maternal and child health nurse, GP or school principal are all likely to provide valuable support and guidance in getting further help if needed.

I'll give you an example from my work in the clinic. Sarah and her four children were sent to see me after a falling out with one of my colleagues, another developmental paediatrician on my team. Sarah had become very upset with that clinician and refused to see them again. I knew that person well, and they were a great clinician, but sometimes we just aren't the right person to form a partnership with a particular family. I was happy to meet Sarah and had the benefit of knowing there was a risk that she might feel like our services were not supporting her. But I still stuffed it up.

Sarah came into the clinic without any of her children the first time I met her. I think she wanted to see what she thought of me before making her kids meet yet another professional who would ask them personal questions that focused on everything they and their mum were doing wrong. Sarah's children were aged from nine to fourteen and all were struggling with emotional and behavioural difficulties. Only the nine-year-old was able to attend school, because the three older children had all been expelled due to violence and property damage. Mia, the nine-year-old, was also on track for expulsion if her behaviour at school didn't improve.

Sarah had fled domestic violence a year prior and was being supported by a number of community services, including child protection. She was so apprehensive of me that at first she only gave me single-word answers. I could tell she didn't want to be there, but she also knew her children might be removed from her care if she didn't comply with the services. What an awful situation to be in, I thought as I talked with her about how I might be able to help.

I could relate, as I grew up in a similar home to Sarah's. My mum was frequently stressed and overwhelmed. Yelling, fighting and hostility were common experiences growing up. My mum was completely alone in dealing with her own mental illness for many years. She was severely depressed but saw no other option than to keep pushing through to provide for her three boys. If there was one thing I could change about my past, it would be to go back and find a way to give her the help she needed. Selfishly, I think it would have made a massive difference to my own mental health, too.

I could tell that Sarah didn't trust me, and she had no reason to. One thing I've learnt about trying to restore trust is to acknowledge what has happened and call out the need to repair it. 'I know that our service has let you down, Sarah,' I said. 'Do you feel comfortable telling me what happened?'

She tensed up, but then decided to talk. 'None of you listen.

There is something wrong with my kids, but no one actually wants to help. That last bloke just nodded and then told me I need to listen to my kids more. What a joke. None of you listen to me!'

I apologised for what she'd experienced and said I wanted to listen to her and understand how I could help. I also asked her what I could do to fix what had happened between her and our service. 'Sort my kids out and get child protection off my back' was the answer that came back to me. While I would word them differently, I agreed with both of those goals. Improving things for her four children and no longer requiring the involvement of child protection were what I was hoping for too.

I asked what was going on for her kids. 'They constantly fight at home, disrespect me and lie. The two oldest are always hiding stuff from me. School got sick of them and said they can't come back until someone sorts them out. I've been trying to get help for years, but no one actually cares. Then my second youngest got kicked out of school and now my youngest is on the same track. I may as well just give up and let child protection have them.'

When I asked what Sarah thought was the cause of the kids struggling so much, she said she had no idea. She'd tried punishments but they didn't work. She ended up in a screaming match with them every night to get off their devices, eat dinner and then get to bed. Most nights she gave up and just let them do what they wanted. When I asked who helped her, she said no one. She had left home as a teenager and didn't have any contact with her parents or siblings. The children's father wasn't allowed to see them or her, and she had no friends in the new town she had been relocated to by services to protect her from her ex-partner.

I asked if anyone at school had been helpful. I knew the wellbeing team at the school the children attended and how fantastic they were. 'They said they were going to help, but once Brayden, my eldest, started hitting other kids and teachers they changed their tune.' I asked about Rebecca and Jennifer, the two wellbeing leads at the school. 'Oh, they were nice, but never helpful.'

Always ask

There is an important distinction between being kind and being helpful. Kindness is an essential part of forming a partnership with people, especially those who have had negative experiences, but it doesn't mean you're helping. A colleague of mine asked me how I knew if I was helping parents. I replied that I could tell from their body language, tone of voice, facial expressions and the fact that they kept coming back to see me in the clinic. I could tell that wasn't the answer he was looking for, so I asked him how he knew he was helping people. 'I ask them.' That simple answer changed the way I work with families.

At the second appointment, Sarah brought all four kids in. It was fairly chaotic in the room but a good opportunity to observe their interactions. Straight from the beginning, the kids were playing up, pushing each other's buttons and ignoring Sarah's attempts to get them to settle down. 'You see what I mean? They don't listen to me,' Sarah said. She explained that things had been challenging since her first child was born. She wasn't aware that she was pregnant with Brayden until quite late and the pregnancy was very challenging. Her partner was a drug addict, and Sarah had been using until she found out she was pregnant. Brayden was little when he was born and didn't feed well. He was also really unsettled and slept poorly. She told me this never improved and even now he hardly ate or slept.

The next child, Ethan, was struggling even more. He'd needed to be admitted to hospital because he wasn't putting on any weight. That was when child protection first became involved, as there were concerns about drug use and violence in the home. It was only after two more children and ten years that Dane, Sarah's partner, was finally arrested and charged for assault against her. During the rest of the appointment, I heard about the behavioural difficulties of all of the children in early childcare and then school, which were the same behaviours Sarah was struggling with at home. They caused so much disruption and risk in the classroom that three of the four kids were not able to attend again until they had been assessed by a specialist.

I needed to go through that assessment for each child, but there was a more pressing issue I needed to get to first: Sarah's mental health. I could see she was completely drowning in stress and hopelessness, but unfortunately she didn't see it that way. 'I'm fine. I just need all of you to do your job.'

In a situation like Sarah's, I usually take things very slowly and try to find the specific motivation for a parent to engage with adult mental health services and then help them to see the benefit. With Sarah, though, I failed at this. I knew she had been offered mental health services many times in the past but had always refused. She had become so used to the behavioural difficulties in her children that she only saw two options for addressing them. The first was to escalate along with them and use hostility and punishments to try to gain their compliance. The second was to ignore them. Both options simply increased the unwanted behaviour in her children. Understandably, her own trauma and mental illness meant that ignoring them was often the best of the two choices.

Unfortunately, the absence of parental guidance in the early years had left all of the children to fend for themselves in managing their emotions. I'm sure educators and other professionals had tried to turn things around, but the home environment meant that those efforts were unsuccessful. Just because Sarah had her own trauma to deal with did not mean that her parenting approaches would be ineffective. I've seen so many parents go through trauma and mental illness and still provide unconditional love, support and guidance to children. But the combination of her poor mental health and not knowing how to help her kids was perpetuating the negative cycles they were stuck in.

Over time I thought I had formed a partnership with Sarah and found the motivation to address her own mental health needs. In reality, it was her new child protection worker who really helped her turn a corner. The previous worker had become burnt out and left the profession. It's a common story: child protection professionals are so overburdened and under resourced that many of them don't last in the job. The new worker was named Melissa and she drove me crazy. She would call or email me with demands that needed to be met that day. She didn't care how busy I was, I needed to contact this person, fill out this form or find a sooner appointment to see Sarah and the kids.

Even though I found it frustrating at times, I always did what Melissa asked, because I knew she only wanted the best for Sarah and her kids, and they were the family I was the most worried about at that time. Melissa was the only one getting anywhere with them. I certainly wasn't. It was only after a couple of months of working with Melissa that Sarah finally went and saw someone. I'm sure the impact of seeing how hard Melissa worked for her and the kids was a big part of it. Also, Melissa was from her community, and they shared a great deal of life experiences. With time, it came out that Sarah had been abused as a child and never wanted her own kids fearing she would unintentionally traumatise them too. She talked about her concerns that her own struggles and lack of confidence being a parent would have consequences on them, just as her mum hadn't been able to protect her. Dane had insisted that she have children, but his violence, drug use and physical abuse only increased after they were born. If it wasn't for the police showing up one night, she wasn't sure that she would still be alive.

It will never cease to amaze me how some people can keep going after experiencing such pain. My work in the clinic is a great reminder of how resilient people can be.

With time, Sarah accepted that working on her own mental health was worthwhile, and we were able to help her get the support and treatment she needed. The children were assessed and diagnosed with a number of neurodevelopmental conditions. They also received treatment for their trauma through counselling and working with their educators to build their capacity through trauma-informed practice. Sarah was also diagnosed with ADHD and found life much easier once she got some help with managing that. Appointments with the kids are still chaotic, and I think they always will be. I don't care though. Seeing Sarah enjoying her children, confident in her own parenting and on the path to recovery is all that really matters.

Key lessons from Chapter 10:

- Parenting children can be an overwhelming experience that can contribute to mental illness, disconnection and a reduced ability to provide the care our children need. Proactively nurturing our own mental health or taking steps to improve when we realise we're struggling is often the first step in any strategy.
- Supporting children who are struggling places great demands on us mentally, and it can bring up difficulties we experienced in childhood where we may not have been supported in the best way possible. While this can motivate us to do better for our own children, it can lead to difficult emotions and reduce our capacity to help others. The first step in addressing this is being aware of it and its influence on our responses. The second is to seek support to improve our own emotional difficulties.
- As adults supporting children, we need to openly demonstrate our own struggles with mental health and, more importantly, how we address these in our daily lives. This shows our kids that challenges are a part of life and lets us model the practical ways we address our own mental health needs. This increases the likelihood that our children will feel safe in expressing and seeking support for their own emotional struggles. It also

gives us greater capacity to meet the demands placed upon us and succeed in our parenting journey, the most important part of which is providing unconditional love and support.

Strategies for parents:

- All adults supporting children need to prioritise their own wellbeing. It increases their capacity to continue to support the kids they care for and models how important this is for them too.
- When supporting a child overwhelms us, it is easy to think the solution sits with the child – if they change, so will our situation. While there is often a need to guide the child to healthier and more appropriate behaviours, this rarely happens quickly and is never the entire answer.
- Instead, we should think about the impact these challenges are having on us and the feelings they bring up about our own childhood, self-esteem and relationships. Many people need the support of a clinician to go through this process. When we understand this, we open up huge potential growth for us personally and for the loved ones in our life.

Afterword

In this book, I have tried to show how we can apply the evidence of child development in practical ways to support the emotional and social skills of our kids. How we respond to emotions is one of the most difficult things to model as parents, because our own emotions are so closely tied to our children's. In addition, we can mistakenly see our childhood self in our children and provide the support we received or wished we had, rather than focusing on what they actually need. Making sure we are responding to the emotions of the child in front of us is a helpful way to avoid this pitfall.

I've shared the stories of just a handful of the thousands of families I've met in my developmental clinic. It's a beautiful thing to be seen as a source of hope and recovery for children who are struggling. Every day I am humbled by the efforts of caregivers and professionals who are striving to improve the lives of the children they support. I'm a very small part of their lives, and these days I feel like a guide who occasionally pops in to lend a hand, but it's parents and teachers who have the greatest opportunities to make a difference. Families tell me where they are, and then where they want to be. My role is to show them the way, give them some tools and cheer for them when the journey gets tough. I still can't believe I get paid for it.

For many of us who do this work, there is another reward. Our own challenges in childhood led us to want to find ways to improve the experience of other children having a tough time. One universal shared experience connects every single person – we were all children once. Harnessing that can motivate us to be better parents and professionals working in this space, and guide us towards empathy for the children we support. I often think I am so passionate about this work, especially helping the kids who are really struggling, because of my own struggles. Being a part of improving the lives of children helps me to heal my own wounds.

In the dedication of this book, I mentioned that I've written it to help the future generation who will be Yvette and Charlie's peers. We have so much potential in our community for kindness, inclusion and togetherness, but we need to do this better, because too many kids are being left behind. That isolation and lack of connection sets up a vicious cycle that impacts us all, but childhood is when we can catch them and guide them to a better future.

In truth, my work also guides me in how I support my own children. The best parents I've met in the clinic are not flawless or sacrificing everything for their children. They are constantly learning and striving to grow. They are led by their children and adjust how they act, realising that for our kids to improve, often we need to improve first. Instead of spending every minute focused on their children, they make sure that the time they have with them is rich, positive and filled with joy and love. They see the privilege in being a part of these beautiful growing beings and know that their time with them is limited, but the memories we create with them will echo long after we have gone. Those parents guide me, and I hope that in a small way I have helped you to be guided by them too.

Resources

Seeking support

Supporting a child who is struggling can be one of the most challenging experiences that exists for parents, and no one should feel alone in this journey. If the challenges feel too tough or things aren't getting better, then seeking clinical support is really important. Every community is different, but all of them have people working hard to help children and families who are facing difficulties.

Often the first professionals to approach are those at the coalface. Maternal and Child Health Nurses support families in the early years. They are expertly trained in child development and can help navigate the health system if needed. In my experience, they are also compassionate allies who stand beside families on their journey. Educators are the most important professionals in children's lives. They are also increasingly being resourced to connect families to clinical support, and often have a large amount of knowledge about how children are going in their daily lives. Talking with them about your concerns can open up avenues of support. Finally General Practitioners (GPs) are the most important medical specialists we have. All families should proactively build a relationship with a GP that you can call upon during future challenges, and please talk to them if you have identified that you need more support at home.

Books

The Work/Parent Switch: How to parent smarter not harder by Anita Cleare, Random House, 2020.

Brain-Body Parenting: How to stop managing behaviour and start raising joyful, resilient kids by Mona Delahooke, John Murray, 2022.

Growing Up in Public: Coming of age in a digital world by Devorah Heitner, Penguin, 2023.

Discipline Without Damage: How to get your kids to behave without messing them up by Vanessa Lapointe, Greystone Books, 2016.

The 5 Principles of Parenting: Your essential guide to raising good humans by Aliza Pressman, Headline Publishing Group, 2024.

Differently Wired: The parent's guide to raising an atypical child by Deborah Reber, Workman, 2020.

The Whole-brain Child: 12 revolutionary strategies to nurture your child's developing mind by Daniel J. Siegel and Tina Payne Bryson, Scribe Publications, 2012.

Websites

Raising Children Network
raisingchildren.net.au

guidinggrowingminds.com

Phone support (in Australia)

Lifeline 13 11 14
Kids Helpline (counselling service for those aged 5 to 25)
1800 551 800

Podcasts

Pop Culture Parenting

References

Introduction

1. Australian Bureau of Statistics. (2022). *Causes of Death, Australia*. ABS. https://www.abs.gov.au/statistics/health/causes-death/causes-death-australia/latest-release.
2. Solmi, M., Radua, J., Olivola, M., Croce, E., Soardo, L., Salazar de Pablo, G., ... & Fusar-Poli, P. (2022). Age at onset of mental disorders worldwide: large-scale meta-analysis of 192 epidemiological studies. *Molecular psychiatry*, 27(1), 281–295.
3. McGorry, P. D., & Mei, C. (2018). Early intervention in youth mental health: progress and future directions. *BMJ Ment Health*, *21*(4), 182–184.
4. Mulraney, M., Lee, C., Freed, G., Sawyer, M., Coghill, D., Sciberras, E., ... & Hiscock, H. (2021). How long and how much? Wait times and costs for initial private child mental health appointments. *Journal of Paediatrics and Child Health*, 57(4), 526–532.

Chapter 1: Attachment

1. Bowlby, J. (1969). *Attachment and loss* (No. 79). Random House.
2. Watson, J. B. (1928). Psychological care of infant and child. WW Norton.
3. Tronick, E. Z. (2018). Emotions and emotional communication in infants. *Parent-infant psychodynamics*, 35–53.
4. Pascalis, O., de Schonen, S., Morton, J., Deruelle, C., & Fabre-Grenet, M. (1995). Mother's face recognition by neonates: A replication and an extension. *Infant behavior and development*, *18*(1), 79–85.
5. Fifer, W. P., & Moon, C. M. (1994). The role of mother's voice in the organization of brain function in the newborn. *Acta paediatrica*, *83*, 86–93.
6. Australian Institute of Health and Welfare. (2012). Perinatal depression: data from the 2010 Australian National Infant Feeding Survey. Canberra: AIHW.
7. Center on the Developing Child at Harvard University (2016). From Best Practices to Breakthrough Impacts: A Science-Based Approach to Building a More Promising Future for Young Children and Families
8. Thomas, A., & Chess, S. (1977). *Temperament and development*. Brunner/Mazel.
9. Wolke, D., Bilgin, A., & Samara, M. (2017). Systematic review and meta-analysis: fussing and crying durations and prevalence of colic in infants. *The Journal of pediatrics*, *185*, 55–61.
10. Freedman, S. B., Al-Harthy, N., & Thull-Freedman, J. (2009). The crying infant: diagnostic testing and frequency

of serious underlying disease. *Pediatrics, 123*(3), 841–848.

11. Bowlby, J. (1969). Attachment and loss. Volume I: Attachment
12. Young, E. S., Simpson, J. A., Griskevicius, V., Huelsnitz, C. O., & Fleck, C. (2019). Childhood attachment and adult personality: A life history perspective. *Self and Identity, 18*(1), 22–38.
13. Bremner, J. G., Slater, A. M., & Johnson, S. P. (2015). Perception of object persistence: The origins of object permanence in infancy. *Child Development Perspectives, 9*(1), 7–13.
14. Strathearn, L., Li, J., Fonagy, P., & Montague, P. R. (2008). What's in a smile? Maternal brain responses to infant facial cues. *Pediatrics, 122*(1), 40–51.
15. Zeanah, C. H., Egger, H. L., Smyke, A. T., Nelson, C. A., Fox, N. A., Marshall, P. J., & Guthrie, D. (2009). Institutional rearing and psychiatric disorders in Romanian preschool children. *American Journal of Psychiatry, 166*(7), 777–785.
16. Cook, F., Giallo, R., Hiscock, H., Mensah, F., Sanchez, K., & Reilly, S. (2019). Infant regulation and child mental health concerns: a longitudinal study. *Pediatrics, 143*(3).

Chapter 2: Behaviour

1. Hoffenaar, P., & Overbeek, G. (2022). Temper tantrums in toddlers and preschoolers: Longitudinal associations with adjustment problems. *Journal of Developmental & Behavioral Pediatrics, 43*(7), 409–417.

Chapter 3: Social skills

1. Metzler, M., Merrick, M. T., Klevens, J., Ports, K. A., & Ford, D. C. (2017). Adverse childhood experiences and life opportunities: Shifting the narrative. *Children and youth services review, 72*, 141–149.
2. Meltzoff, A. N., & Moore, M. K. (1977). Imitation of facial and manual gestures by human neonates. *Science, 198*(4312), 75–78.
3. Swain, J. E., Lorberbaum, J. P., Kose, S., & Strathearn, L. (2007). Brain basis of early parent–infant interactions: psychology, physiology, and in vivo functional neuroimaging studies. *Journal of child psychology and psychiatry, and allied disciplines, 48*, 262.
4. Weiner, I. B., Lerner, R. M., Easterbrooks, M. A., & Mistry, J. (2012). *Handbook of psychology, developmental psychology* (Vol. 6). John Wiley & Sons.
5. Piaget, J. (1926). *The language and thought of the children.* New York: Turbner and Co., Ltd.
6. Eisenberg, Nancy, Tracy L. Spinrad, and Amanda S. Morris, (2013) 'Prosocial Development', in Philip David Zelazo (ed.), *The Oxford Handbook of Developmental Psychology, Vol. 2: Self and Other*, Oxford Library of Psychology.
7. Mann, M., Hosman, C. M., Schaalma, H. P., & De Vries, N. K. (2004). Self-esteem in a broad-spectrum approach for mental health promotion. *Health education research, 19*(4), 357–372.
8. Gunnar, M. R., & Herrera, A. M. (2013). The development of stress reactivity: A neurobiological perspective. *The Oxford handbook of developmental psychology*, 2, 45–80.
9. Owens, Robert E., Jr.. *Language Development : An Introduction*,

Pearson Education, (2019). *ProQuest Ebook Central*, https://ebookcentral.proquest.com/lib/unimelb/detail.action?docID=5894757.

10. Hart, B., Risley, T. R., & Kirby, J. R. (1997). Meaningful differences in the everyday experience of young American children. *Canadian Journal of Education*, 22(3), 323.
11. Crowe, B., Machalicek, W., Wei, Q., Drew, C., & Ganz, J. (2022). Augmentative and alternative communication for children with intellectual and developmental disability: A mega-review of the literature. *Journal of developmental and physical disabilities*, 1–42.

Chapter 4: Emotional development

1. Ardoin, N. M., & Bowers, A. W. (2020). Early childhood environmental education: A systematic review of the research literature. *Educational Research Review, 31*, 100353.
2. Boyce, W. T. (2019). *The orchid and the dandelion: Why sensitive people struggle and how all can thrive*. Pan MacMillan.
3. Menting, A. T., de Castro, B. O., & Matthys, W. (2013). Effectiveness of the Incredible Years parent training to modify disruptive and prosocial child behavior: A meta-analytic review. *Clinical psychology review*, 33(8), 901–913.

Chapter 5: Self-esteem

1. Friedman, S. L., & Scholnick, E. K. (2022). Theories of Human Development1. *Developmental-Behavioral Pediatrics E-Book*, 19.
2. Orenstein, G. A., & Lewis, L. (2022). Eriksons stages of psychosocial development. In *StatPearls [Internet]*. StatPearls Publishing.

3. Rubin, K. H., & Chronis-Tuscano, A. (2021). Perspectives on social withdrawal in childhood: Past, present, and prospects. *Child development perspectives*, *15*(3), 160–167.
4. Orth, U., & Robins, R. W. (2022). Is high self-esteem beneficial? Revisiting a classic question. *American Psychologist*, *77*(1), 5.
5. Dweck, C. S. (2013). Social development. *The Oxford handbook of developmental psychology*, 2, 167–90.
6. Loyer Carbonneau, M., Demers, M., Bigras, M., & Guay, M. C. (2021). Meta-analysis of sex differences in ADHD symptoms and associated cognitive deficits. *Journal of Attention Disorders*, *25*(12), 1640–1656.
7. Thomas, R., Sanders, S., Doust, J., Beller, E., & Glasziou, P. (2015). Prevalence of attention-deficit/hyperactivity disorder: a systematic review and meta-analysis. *Pediatrics*, *135*(4), e994-e1001.
8. Association, A. P. (2013). *Diagnostic and statistical manual of mental disorders: 5th edn.*
9. ADHD Guideline Development Group. (2022). Australian evidence-based clinical practice guideline for Attention Deficit Hyperactivity. Melbourne: Australasian ADHD Professionals Association.
10. Best, J. R., & Miller, P. H. (2010). A developmental perspective on executive function. *Child development*, *81*(6), 1641–1660.
11. Orth, U., & Robins, R. W. (2014). The development of self-esteem. *Current directions in psychological science*, 23(5), 381–387.

Chapter 6: Anxiety

1. Kessler, R. C., Avenevoli, S., McLaughlin, K. A., Green, J. G., Lakoma, M. D., Petukhova, M., … & Merikangas, K. R. (2012). Lifetime co-morbidity of DSM-IV disorders in the US national comorbidity survey replication adolescent supplement (NCS-A). *Psychological medicine*, 42(9), 1997–2010.
2. GBD 2019 Mental Disorders Collaborators. (2022). Global, regional, and national burden of 12 mental disorders in 204 countries and territories, 1990–2019: a systematic analysis for the Global Burden of Disease Study 2019. *The Lancet Psychiatry*, 9(2), 137–150.
3. Lawrence, D., Johnson, S., Hafekost, J., Boterhoven de Haan, K., Sawyer, M., Ainley, J., & Zubrick, S. R. (2015). The mental health of children and adolescents: Report on the second Australian child and adolescent survey of mental health and wellbeing.
4. Muris, P., & Ollendick, T. H. (2021). Current challenges in the diagnosis and management of selective mutism in children. *Psychology Research and Behavior Management*, 159–167.
5. Rosenberg DR, Chiriboga JA. (2020) Anxiety disorders. In: Kliegman RM, St. Geme JW, Blum NJ, Shah SS, Tasker RC, Wilson KM, eds. *Nelson Textbook of Pediatrics*. 21st ed.
6. Hofmann, S. G., Asnaani, A., Vonk, I. J., Sawyer, A. T., & Fang, A. (2012). The efficacy of cognitive behavioral therapy: A review of meta-analyses. *Cognitive therapy and research*, 36, 427–440.
7. Critchley, H. D., & Garfinkel, S. N. (2017). Interoception and emotion. *Current opinion in psychology*, 17, 7–14.

Chapter 7: Respect

1. Wellman, H. M. (2017). The development of theory of mind: Historical reflections. *Child Development Perspectives*, *11*(3), 207–214.
2. Tomasello, M., & Haberl, K. (2003). Understanding attention: 12-and 18-month-olds know what is new for other persons. *Developmental psychology*, *39*(5), 906.
3. Astington, Janet Wilde, and Claire Hughes. (2013). 'Theory of Mind: Self-Reflection and Social Understanding', in Philip David Zelazo (ed.), *The Oxford Handbook of Developmental Psychology, Vol. 2: Self and Other*, Oxford Library of Psychology
4. Wellman H. M., Cross D., & Watson J. (2001). Meta-analysis of theory of mind development: The truth about false-belief. *Child Development*, 72, 655–684.
5. Wimmer H., & Perner J. (1983). Beliefs about beliefs: Representation and constraining function of wrong beliefs in young children's understanding of deception. *Cognition*, 13, 103–128.
6. Astington, Janet Wilde, and Claire Hughes. (2013).
7. Dweck, C. S. (2013). Social development. *The Oxford handbook of developmental psychology*, 2, 167–90.

Chapter 8: Depression

1. Walter H. & DeMaso D. (2020) 'Mood Disorders' in Richard E. Behrman, Robert M. Kliegman, Hal B. Jenson. (2000). *Nelson textbook of pediatrics.*
2. GBD 2019 Mental Disorders Collaborators. (2022). Global, regional, and national burden of 12 mental disorders in 204 countries and territories, 1990–2019: a systematic analysis

for the Global Burden of Disease Study 2019. *The Lancet Psychiatry*, *9*(2), 137–150.

3. Monroe, S. M., & Harkness, K. L. (2011). Recurrence in major depression: a conceptual analysis. *Psychological review*, *118*(4), 655.
4. American Psychiatric Association. (2013). *Diagnostic and statistical manual of mental disorders: 5th Edn*.
5. Berg, K. L., Shiu, C. S., Acharya, K., Stolbach, B. C., & Msall, M. E. (2016). Disparities in adversity among children with autism spectrum disorder: a population-based study. Developmental Medicine & Child Neurology, 58(11), 1124–1131; and Brown, N. M., Brown, S. N., Briggs, R. D., Germán, M., Belamarich, P. F., & Oyeku, S. O. (2017). Associations between adverse childhood experiences and ADHD diagnosis and severity. *Academic pediatrics*, *17*(4), 349–355.
6. Swannell, S. V., Martin, G. E., Page, A., Hasking, P., & St John, N. J. (2014). Prevalence of nonsuicidal self-injury in nonclinical samples: Systematic review, meta-analysis and meta-regression. *Suicide and Life-Threatening Behavior*, 44(3), 273–303.
7. Nock, M. K., Green, J. G., Hwang, I., McLaughlin, K. A., Sampson, N. A., Zaslavsky, A. M., & Kessler, R. C. (2013). Prevalence, correlates, and treatment of lifetime suicidal behavior among adolescents: results from the National Comorbidity Survey Replication Adolescent Supplement. *JAMA psychiatry*, 70(3), 300–310.
8. Park, R. J., & Goodyer, I. M. (2000). Clinical guidelines for depressive disorders in childhood and adolescence. *European child & adolescent psychiatry*, 9, 147–161.

Chapter 9: 'Bad' kids

1. Ogundele, M. O. (2018). Behavioural and emotional disorders in childhood: A brief overview for paediatricians. *World journal of clinical pediatrics*, 7(1), 9.
2. Burke, J. D., Rowe, R., & Boylan, K. (2014). Functional outcomes of child and adolescent oppositional defiant disorder symptoms in young adult men. *Journal of child psychology and psychiatry*, 55(3), 264–272.
3. Bornstein, M. H. (2012). Cultural approaches to parenting. *Parenting, 12*(2–3), 212–221.
4. Lunkenheimer, E., Lichtwarck-Aschoff, A., Hollenstein, T., Kemp, C. J., & Granic, I. (2016). Breaking down the coercive cycle: How parent and child risk factors influence real-time variability in parental responses to child misbehavior. *Parenting*, 16(4), 237–256.

Chapter 10: You

1. Pinquart, M. (2017). Associations of parenting dimensions and styles with externalizing problems of children and adolescents: An updated meta-analysis. *Developmental psychology*, 53(5), 873.

Acknowledgements

This book has only been possible thanks to the unconditional support from my amazing wife, Annaliese. She believes in the vision that the book and my other advocacy work hopes to achieve. Despite working even more than I do, she takes the lion's share of supporting our family. Without her, I would be very limited in my ability to help others.

Second, I must thank the families and professionals who I've worked with and learnt from over the last twenty-plus years. This book is my attempt to share with others what you've taught me. The following are people who have directly supported this journey. They have generously given their time, expertise and perspective to strengthen the goal of improving the lives of children around the world: Kevin Anderson, Tim Bartley, Hamish Blake, Miffany Blythe, Anita Cleare, Mona Delahooke, Maggie Dent, Daryl Efron, Joshua Feder, Eddie Geller, Adam Gregory, Sarah Harden, Devorah Heitner, Sam Jockel, Henri Jones, Evan Kaldor, Vanessa Lapointe,

Nick McCormack, Hamish McLachlan, Rob Moodie, Carmen Myler, Tina Payne Bryson, Brooke Perry (and the AV1 team), Bruce Perry, Aliza Pressman, Deborah Reber, Terri Scanlon, Dan Siegel, Nick Speer, Nick Stone, Hugh van Cuylenburg, Mark Vickers-Willis, Michael Wipfli and Lyndelle Zuccolin.

I must also thank my wonderful literary agent, Tara Wynne of Curtis Brown, and my editors Sophie Ambrose, Amanda Martin and Brandon VanOver of Penguin Random House. I never intended to write a book, but both Tara and Sophie believed in the project before I did. The expertise and support of all four has been essential to create a piece of work that hopes to guide those supporting children.